**Marion Stanton** is the 40 year old mother of three children, including Danny who has cerebral palsy. She is a qualified special needs teacher and is currently studying for a Masters in Education with the Open University. She has previously worked in occupational therapy and housing. Since becoming a parent of a disabled child Marion has co-founded a parent-run early learning group for child          disabilities and has been an active member of the A          Inclusive Education which campaigns for the righ*          hildren and young people to be educated in the          also been involved in conferences on comm          disabled children.

# THE
# Cerebral Palsy
# HANDBOOK

## A practical guide
## for parents and carers

## Marion Stanton

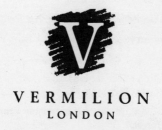

VERMILION
LONDON

This book is dedicated to Danny Stanton, his brother Tam, his sister Katie, his grandad, Edgar Wille and to the memory of Molly.

First published 1992 by Optima

1 3 5 7 9 10 8 6 4 2

Copyright © 1992, 1997 Marion Stanton

This edition published in the United Kingdom in 1997 by Vermilion, an imprint of Ebury Press

Random House UK Ltd
Random House
20 Vauxhall Bridge Road
London SW1V 2SA

Random House Australia (Pty) Ltd
20 Alfred Street, Milsons Point, Sydney,
New South Wales 2061, Australia

Random House, New Zealand Limited
18 Poland Rd, Glenfield,
Auckland 10, New Zealand

Random House, South Africa (Pty) Limited
Endulini, 5A Jubilee Road,
Parktown 2193, South Africa

Random House UK Limited Reg. No. 954009

A CIP catalogue record for this book is available from the British Library.

ISBN 0 09 181507 X

Typeset in 10½ pt Palatino by Deltatype Ltd, Birkenhead, Merseyside
Printed and bound in Great Britain by MacKays of Chatham, plc

Papers used by Vermilion are natural, recyclable products made from wood grown in sustainable forests.

# CONTENTS

# FOREWORD

The discovery that your child has cerebral palsy can be a bewildering and devastating experience. Medical and other professionals may appear distant and vague in their explanations. Textbooks seem obscure, old-fashioned and unhelpful. Advice from different experts is frequently impractical or downright contradictory. There doesn't seem to be any co-ordinated source of information and practical help.

Marion Stanton has seen the need at first hand, and has produced a book that tackles the issues head-on. This is not an academic book written by a dispassionate observer. It is a book written from the inside, from personal experience of the problems of a parent of a child with cerebral palsy. It's practical, down-to-earth and packed with useful information. Like Marion Stanton, I believe that the parents of a child with cerebral palsy are the single most important source of input, support and therapy. This book aims to help parents to be better equipped. It deserves to be read.

John Wyatt BSc, MBBS, MRCP, DCH
Consultant Paediatrician
University College Hospital

# PREFACE

I was much too tired and confused to take in the full implications of Danny's condition in the first couple of months of his life. I had had a relatively normal pregnancy but then, at the onset of labour, I suddenly started to bleed heavily. I was rushed into hospital and Danny was born by emergency caesarean section 40 minutes after I had dialled 999. He was not breathing at all when he was lifted out and it took a full eight minutes for the medical team to resuscitate him. He was then rushed into intensive care where he was put immediately onto a respirator and given heavy doses of barbiturates to control the massive fits that he was having.

The first I knew of all this was shortly after I came round in the labour ward. I was given a private room off the main post-natal ward. During those first couple of days numerous kind faces above blue or white coats would appear periodically at my bedside and attempt to explain what was happening. I heard the words but they didn't seem to mean anything. Eventually I was well enough to go down to the special care unit and see my baby. He was lying absolutely still. It was only later that I discovered his lack of movement was due to drugs as much as to his condition. Several quiet counselling sessions in a room specially set aside for the purpose finally got the message across that Danny might be brain damaged.

When Danny was about 4 months old, and after constant badgering, I managed to get a diagnosis out of his consultant at the hospital. He has severe, spastic, cerebral palsy. The consultant stressed that it was not always so easy to give a diagnosis at such an early stage but that in Danny's case the symptoms were obvious.

Not all children with cerebral palsy enter the world as violently as Danny did. In some cases it dawns on parents gradually, possibly over a period of many months, that there is something not quite right with their child. Many will share their concerns with their general practitioner, to be judged as worriers and sent home with assurances that 'some babies develop later than others', only to discover, finally, that their intuition was right all along.

By the time Danny was 6 months old we had established a routine which included regular home visits from numerous therapists and plentiful trips to the hospital. I went back to work and was lucky enough to find someone, who later became a very good friend, who wanted to care for him while I was at work. We very quickly became frustrated by the lack of co-ordination, information and practical support available to families when one of their members has cerebral palsy. There seems to be plenty of opportunity to talk about these frustrations and to get hold of a sympathetic ear from one or another of the therapists or health visitors arriving regularly on the doorstep but very little in the way of practical help in the form of money, childcare or even contacts through whom we might be able to get information.

My current concern is to get Danny sufficient services to enable him to stay in a mainstream school with his sister. The obstacles and lack of information in this respect are equally, if not more, difficult to get hold of than early medical advice. I am now beginning to realise the far reaching effects which professionals, who only see your child for a very short space of time before they write reports on their ability and potential, can have on a child's chance of having a full and equal place in society. I find it incredibly sad that much of the energy which should be joyfully put into helping my child to enjoy his life is expended on a seemingly never ending battle for access to services and facilities to which he has a right.

Most of the understanding I have gained of the options available has been through chance (such as bumping into someone who happened to know about conductive education) and by investigations resembling detective work.

It is for this reason that I have decided to write this book. I hope that it will give other families the opportunity to scan some of the alternatives, get a better understanding of cerebral palsy and make positive choices.

I am not a qualified doctor nor a therapist. I am writing this book as a parent for other parents. I believe (and many professionals share this belief) that a child with cerebral palsy's best therapist is the person who cares for her on a day to day basis. The role of the health and education professionals is to support the family in helping the child to reach her full potential.

Prior to having Danny I spent some time working in various

aspects of the health service and extensively in the housing field, as well as taking an Open University degree which focused on psychology and social sciences. I am now a qualified teacher working with children who need extra support with their learning. I'm sure that these experiences have contributed to the style of the book but I hope that I have managed to produce a publication which is easily accessible to all carers of children with cerebral palsy. I have done my best to steer away from the 'academic' and the 'clinical'.

Wherever possible I have tried to use language that anyone can understand. I have been extremely irritated by the text books about cerebral palsy which really can be understood only by professional people. I hope that this book will be more accessible.

When discussing people who do not have a disability I use the term 'non-disabled' rather than the currently fashionable 'able bodied'. The intention is to move even further away from the tendency those without a disability may have to see themselves as 'normal' and those with a disability as 'not normal'.

The pronouns 'she' and 'he' are used interchangeably throughout the book, unless I am referring to a specific individual.

# ACKNOWLEDGEMENTS

So many people have helped to make this book possible. My apologies if I have missed anyone out.

Thanks for inspiring the idea in the first place to Andrew Wille, Edgar Wille and Andrew Lisiki.

Thanks for help with the research to The Islington Disablement Association, Valerie Hammond, The Spastics Society, Mike Devenney, Eunice Hawkins, Linda Shingler, Sheila Murray, Chris Meadows, Jan Aldous, Preethi Manuel, Gloria Pahad, Tandie Makiwani, Margaret and Trevor from The Kerland Clinic, Andrew Sutton from the Foundation for Conductive Education. The Hornsey Centre for Children Learning, Susan Haughsbrough from the Bobath Centre, Hillary Caime from Richard Cloudsley Primary School, Maria from the Rosemary Primary School, Gavin Evans, Lorna Mighty, Islington MENCAP, Kim Holt, Niki Green, Sarah Laing, Sarah Barnett, Rahila Gupta, Lyn Weeks, Tony Ingram, Scot Hall, Mitchelin Mason, Richard Reiser, Gloria Pahad and Midge Caryer, and Ian, the Head of Springfield School.

Thanks for general back up to Linda and Lorna Evans, Kath Loader, Marianne Verner-Jensen, Isa Nyborg, Anne-Mette Svenstrup, Sally White, Melanie Gore, Sonia Gogna, Nilofar Prentis, Tom Barwood.

Special thanks to John Wyatt, who offered time in his very busy schedule to help with the medical sections, to Andrew Prentis and to Richenda Milton-Thompson for her sensitive editing.

Thanks to the following for their help on the second edition: Margaret Baber, Preethi Manuel, Scope, James Ware and Diana Simpson.

Finally, thanks on my own behalf and that of my readers to Andrew, Jacqueline and Martin for having the generosity of spirit to share their experiences in Chapter 10.

'My life is not really very different from how non-disabled people feel about themselves. It's simply that they wear a cloak of normality, a concept which renders me naked.'

'We both live in the shadow of stereotype. I'm simply lucky enough to be on the fringe, rejected by the stereotype, forced to forge my own identity, my own reality, and to create it anew . . . beautiful, proud and disabled.'

Mary Duffy

# INTRODUCTION

Perhaps one of the most striking features of cerebral palsy is that no two people who have the condition will be the same. Cerebral palsy (or CP as it is often referred to) is one of the most varied medical conditions which exist. It can affect those who have it very mildly so that you would hardly notice they had a disability. It can be moderate, in which case you would be likely to notice the unsteady movements or stiffness of limb but the person who has the CP would still be able to go about his daily life with minimal help. It can be very severe so that the person is unable to move at all. There are many shades in between these three presentations of CP. This variability makes learning about the condition, diagnosing the condition, treating the condition and making outcome predictions extremely difficult.

Cerebral palsy affects children, often from birth, and persists for life. One of the most difficult aspects of CP is that it is hard to know in a child's early years whether she will grow up with mild, moderate or severe cerebral palsy. The extent of her disability unfolds as she grows. These factors contribute enormously to the confusion and frustration often felt by carers who are trying to do their best to give their child a positive start in life.

## What is cerebral palsy?

Cerebral palsy (CP) is *a disorder of movement*. The term relates to the physical condition of a person who has difficulty either producing movement, preventing movement or controlling movement following injury to the brain before or during birth or in the first five years of life. The physical problems presented by cerebral palsy are often referred to as *motor* problems.

The response to injury of the mature or developed brain is quite different from that of the immature or still developing brain. Implications for outcome and treatment are also different from those for cerebral palsy.

A child with CP may also have additional disabilities such as visual or hearing problems, language delay or co-ordination difficulties.

There is no cure for cerebral palsy. Damaged brain cells cannot regenerate. However, there are many ways in which the effects of brain damage may be brought under control so that the individual can live a more fulfilling life than might otherwise have been the case. Doctors are often reluctant to diagnose cerebral palsy when a child is newly showing signs which lead them to suspect it. There may be a number of reasons for this:

- It is not always easy to identify (especially in the very young baby) and doctors are wary of misinforming parents.
- Even when a child has clearly sustained damage to the brain or starts to show signs of having cerebral palsy there are numerous instances of symptoms disappearing leaving the child free of any motor problems and not apparently disabled.
- There are wide variations in the severity of the condition so parents may misinterpret minor problems as being very severe.
- Doctors may exercise caution in informing parents of their suspicions because they fear that the parent will be unable to cope with the information.

# What causes cerebral palsy?

The brain damage may be due to one of a number of factors. Up to 50 per cent of cases of CP have no known cause at present. The following are some of the most common known causes.

## *Prenatal causes (before birth)*

**Haemorrhage (**bleeding)   Haemorrhage in a specific area of the brain is a common cause with premature children who develop cerebral palsy.

**Infection**   Infection may be passed from mother to child in the womb. An example of this is the passing on of cytomegalo-virus (CMV) to the unborn child. The virus is a harmless member of the herpes family but can (in a very small number of cases) cause brain damage to a child if passed to him during pregnancy. German measles (rubella) is a more commonly known virus which can be passed to the child in the womb and cause brain damage.

**Environmental factors** By this I mean that the mother can be affected by something she eats or drinks, or by breathing dangerous poisons in the air, which can be passed on to the child before birth. A recent and famous example of this is a number of children who were born with cerebral palsy after their mothers had eaten cheese containing listeria. Toxoplasmosis is an infection which may be acquired from eating raw or undercooked meat, from cats or from contact with contaminated soil. The infection can then be passed on to the unborn child. Radiation received by the mother (for example through radiotherapy) can also affect the unborn child. There have been a number of specific incidents where the number of children affected in certain geographical areas increased temporarily due to environmental pollution. An epidemic of CP occurred in Minamata Bay, Japan, between 1953 and 1971. This was eventually found to be related to methyl mercury in fish which had been consumed by pregnant women. The discharge of methyl mercury had come from a vinyl chloride acetaldehyde plant.

**Heredity** There has recently been speculation that a small number of cases may be hereditary but there is little evidence to back this up.

## Perinatal causes (at or around the time of birth)

**Lack of oxygen to the brain (asphyxia)** This is a common cause in cases where there are such difficulties at birth as, for example, the umbilical cord being wrapped round the child's neck, the mother haemorrhaging before the baby has been safely delivered, or contractions which are so severe that the supply of oxygen from the placenta is reduced. In these cases the brain damage is often global (involving all of the brain rather than a specific area).

## Postnatal cause (in the first five years of life)

**Head injury** Head injuries sustained during the first five years of life may cause CP.

**Infections** Contracted in early life such as meningitis.

**Lack of oxygen** CP can also be caused by the brain being deprived of oxygen for a period of time due to accident or choking during the first five years of life. A near miss cot death or a near drowning inhalation can have the same effect.

# Different types of CP

The way in which a child's movement is affected will depend on the extent of the brain damage and which areas of the brain are damaged. This is because specific areas of the brain control different motor functions.

A number of attempts have been made to produce classifications of cerebral palsy. Classifications tend to be made either in terms either of the 'type' of CP or of the extent of the disability.

There are four main 'types' of cerebral palsy. These are spastic, athetoid, ataxic and mixed.

## Spastic cerebral palsy (pyramidal)

This is caused by damage to the cortex. The child will be stiff in one or more limbs and possibly all over.

## Athetoid cerebral palsy (extra pyramidal)

Athetoid CP is caused by damage to the basal ganglia (see Figure 1). The child will be floppy in one or more limbs and possibly all over.

## Ataxic cerebral palsy

Ataxic CP is caused by damage to the cerebellum (See Figure 1). The child will be unsteady. Although movement is present it may appear random and bringing these random movements under control may be difficult.

## Mixed cerebral palsy

Mixed is a term used for types of cerebral palsy which do not fit neatly into one of the other three classifications. The child may show signs of more than one type of cerebral palsy.

## Other types

Other, less common, types of cerebral palsy include *dystonia* (where posture distorts intermittently), *chorea* (where fingers and toes jerk spontaneously), *ballismus* (where there is uncontrolled movement of the joints), *rigidity* (where limbs are rigid like lead piping or intermittently resist passive motion), *tremor* and *atonia* (which is similar to athetosis and often develops into it).

## Topographical classification

Cerebral palsy is most commonly classified topographically (in terms of the parts of the body affected and the extent of the disability), as follows:

**Quadriplegia**   All four limbs are affected.

**Diplegia**   All four limbs are affected but the legs more so than the arms. This is common if CP occurs due to a premature birth.

**Paraplegia**   Both legs are affected.

**Triplegia**   Three limbs are affected.

**Hemiplegia**   One side of the body is affected.

**Monoplegia**   One limb is affected.

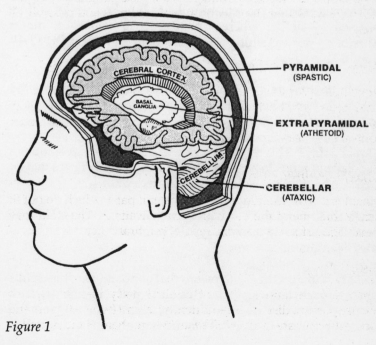

*Figure 1*

## Other common factors

**Additional disabilities**   These may be fairly common and include such problems as difficulty developing speech, difficulty in seeing or difficulty making sense of what is seen (perception), difficulty hearing or difficulty making sense of what is heard, either mild or severe seizures (convulsions or fits), difficulty with the development of understanding and thinking, and learning disorders. Later on there may be difficulty with organising the written word (dyslexia for example). There is also a danger – in certain more severe cases – of muscle contracture (stretching out of shape) and bone deformities.


## Additional terminolgy

Confusion often arises for parents when doctors offer a different diagnosis or use terms which are not immediately identifiable with a known condition.

The following terms (in addition to cerebral palsy and some-times instead of the term) might be used.

**Motor delay**   This means that the child is behind the average in developing normal movement in limbs and body. This will be assessed by noting where a child fails to achieve a 'motor milestone' – such as sitting up by six months or walking by 12–18 months.

**Developmental delay**   This means that the child is behind the average in her motor, vision and fine motor, speech, language and social development.

**Global delay**   This term has a similar meaning to developmental delay but tends to be used where a consultant believes that all aspects of a child's development are affected.

**Intellectually impaired**   This means that the consultant believes the child's understanding to be affected, to an extent which will cause learning difficulties.

**Sensory impairment**   This means that one or more of the child's senses – touch, taste, sight, hearing and smell – are affected.

**Cortical blindness**   Cortical blindness is caused by damage to the cerebral cortex. This means that the child has difficulty making sense of what he sees but it does not necessarily mean that he is blind in the conventional sense. He may be clinically able to see but unable to organise what he sees.

**Multiply handicapped**   This is a general term for children who have several problems of which cerebral palsy may be one.

**Epileptic**   This term is used to describe fits or seizures caused by sudden electrical activity in the brain.

Some children might present with these problems who do not have cerebral palsy and some children who have cerebral palsy also appear to present with one or more of the above.

## Additional questions

### *Is intelligence affected?*

Many carers of children who have cerebral palsy fear that their child may not be intelligent. Intelligence is very complicated and clinical understanding of intelligence is still developing.

The assessment of children's understanding is very difficult when they are young. Tests designed to assess intelligence often require children to have full use of their hands, good hearing and good vision – and may therefore not be appropriate for testing a child who has cerebral palsy. To counter this, therapists will also observe the child's responses to everyday situations. However, these are very difficult to interpret if a child has a problem controlling his movement. Physical disability may inhibit the child's ability to express his mental alertness. In addition to this, assumptions made that a young child is intellectually impaired may lead to his not receiving the appropriate stimulation for his age. This, in turn, could lead to the child failing to develop intellectually to his full capacity but it would be social and environmental factors which were to blame, not the brain damage.

It is impossible to tell whether or not a child who has severe physical problems is also intellectually impaired until the child finds a means of communication with the outside world. This may not happen until the child is 2, 3, or 4 years old or even older in some cases. The family may see signs of a child's understanding well before a consultant does and a consultant may believe that parents over estimate their children's intellectual capabil-

**Table 1** Classification of cerebral palsy, based on the work of Minear (1956) *Paediatrics*, 18(841)

| Physiological (Description by type of movements) | Topographical (Parts of body affected) | Aetiological (Different possible causes) | Incidental factors (Other, non-motor, problems which might arise) |
|---|---|---|---|
| A) Spasticity (stiff) | A) Monoplegia: affects one limb | A) Prenatal (before birth) | A) Intellectual impairment |
| B) Athetosis (floppy) | B) Paraplegia: affects only the legs |   1. Hereditary-genetic | B) Physical state: |
|   1. Tensional (sometimes tense) | C) Hemiplegia: affects one side of |   2. Acquired in the womb: |   1. Small size of body |
|   2. Non-tensional (not tense) |    the body |    (*a*) infection |   2. Developmental delay |
|   3. Dystonic (muscles lack | D) Triplegia: affects three limbs |    (*b*) anoxia (lack of oxygen |   3. Poor bone development |
|    strength) | E) Quadriplegia (tetraplegia): |    (*c*) prenatal cerebral |   4. Contractures: permanent |
|   4. With tremor (muscles quiver) |    affects all four limbs |      haemorrhage |    distortion of muscles |
| C) Rigidity (stiff/no movement) | F) Diplegia: affecting both halves |    (*d*) Rhesus factor | C) Eye and hand movement |
| D) Ataxia (movements irregular |    uniformly: bilateral paralysis |    (*e*) metabolic: inability to | D) Vision: |
|   and jerky) | G) Double hemiplegia; affecting all |      adapt nutrition to service |   1. Sensory loss; damaged cortical |
| E) Tremor |    four limbs but arms more so |      bodily function needs |    area of the brain |
| F) Atonia (rare; muscles lack |    than legs |    (*f*) breech delivery |   2. Motor; control of eye |
|   vigour) | |    (*g*) poor maternal nutrition |    movement or direction |
| G) Mixed (combination of some or | | B) Natal (at birth) |    affected by poor muscle |
|   all of above) | |   1. Anoxia: |    control |
| H) Unclassifiable | |    (*a*) placental failure | E) Hearing: |
| | |    (*b*) drug induced |   1. Loss of pitch |
| | |    (*c*) breech delivery |   2. Loss of decibels |
| | |    (*d*) forceps delivery | F) Speech disorders |
| | |    (*e*) maternal anoxia or | G) Touch: |
| | |      hypotension |   1. Oversensitive |
| | | C) Postnatal (after birth) |   2. Not sensitive |
| | |   1. Accident | H) Taste and smell: |
| | |   2. Infection |   1. Oversensitive |
| | |   3. Poisoning |   2. Not sensitive |
| | |   4. Blood vessel damage | I) Convulsions |
| | |   5. Anoxia | |
| | |   6. Tumour | |

ities because of a strong desire to believe that their children understand. Later on it will be the place of the psychologist and/ or speech and language therapist to assess your child's intellectual capacities. These therapists can contribute very positively by assisting the child to develop early communication.

It used to be believed that intelligence (ability to discriminate and understand numbers and verbal reasoning), cognitive abilities (knowledge), affective behaviour (ability to take action to produce effect) and temperament (personality) were all under the control of the cerebral cortex. It is now believed that these functions are distributed more generally in cortical and subcortical centres. Cases where children appear to have no intellectual and cognitive capacity are very rare if not non-existent.

The kind of terminology which used to be used at the turn of the century and right up until the 1960s in some cases (such as 'mentally defective') have now gone out of everyday use as the negative connotations of such terms have become more generally realised. Many such terms, however, do still exist on legal statute books.

Beliefs about the development of intelligence and the way in which the intelligence is affected in children who have CP have changed radically over the last 100 years. In 1889 Sir William Osler asserted that children with bilateral hemiplegia (now known as spastic quadriplegia) were usually 'imbecile and often idiotic', children with paraplegia offered 'greater hope of mental improvement', a large percentage of children with hemiplegia grew up to be 'feeble minded' and that epilepsy was a 'potent factor in inducing mental deterioration'.

In 1948 Dr Phelps maintained that 30 per cent of persons with cerebral palsy were 'mentally defective' and 70 per cent were 'normal'. Other publications tended to quote the incidence of 'mental deficiency' at around 50 per cent. In the 1950s, Crothers and Paine suggested that the incidence of 'mental deficiency' varied from one category to another of the condition. They maintained that of 80 per cent of 'spastics' with three or more limbs involved, 60 per cent of hemiplegias and 50 per cent of extra-pyramidal cases had an IQ below the average.

In the 1970s Sophie Levitt reported that intelligence varied amongst 'spastics' tending to be lower than in 'athetoids', was frequently good and may be very high in 'athetoids', and was often low in cases of ataxia.

In 1987, Eugene Bleck noted that 'most persons with athetosis have normal intellects and some are superior; children who have spastic diplegia usually succeed in regular school although they may have some specific learning problems; those who have total body involved spastic paralysis [quadriplegia] seem to have a higher incidence of retardation; those with less motor involvement such as ataxia or spastic hemiplegia due to cerebral maldevelopment appear to have more mental retardation.'

I hope this makes it clear that beliefs about the intelligence levels and potential of children who have CP changes over time. Since it is hardly likely that the children's real potential changes we can safely assume that this is a question that the medical profession is not really able to answer on the basis of *type* of CP. It may be that a far more useful approach is to look at ways of maximising a child's learning.

Over recent years some professionals have pioneered a shift of emphasis away from the assumption that intelligence is determined by the extent and type of brain damage and towards a more complex analysis of the development of the intelligence in which many factors (including but not exclusively attributable to brain damage) play a part. Environmental factors are now considered to make a significant contribution to the development of intelligence. In the 1940s, Hebbs maintained that intellectual performance depended on 'cell assembly' developed through repeated stimulation. The notion of the importance of a stimulating environment began to have some prominence.

Lewis Rosenbloom, writing in the 1970s, outlined four different pathways along which children make developmental progress. These are:

- Physical
- Intellectual
- Emotional
- Social

He considered that motor (movement) behaviour acts as a 'linking and integrating mechanism in development'. He and others found that there was a relationship between movement and aspects of intellectual development. He also suggested that motor behaviour contributes to emotional and social development and pointed out that frustration, dependence and lack of social interaction suffered by a child with cerebral palsy increases the likelihood of emotional disturbance and psychiatric disorder. He proposed that programmes should be devised to ensure that children gain motor experience which is aimed at promoting overall development rather than being specific to a child's physical difficulties.

It appears therefore that our intellectual abilities are affected by many inputs and it may be inferred that it is not possible to predict or assume intelligence levels in children who have cerebral palsy as the acquisition of intelligence is determined by many factors external to the child as well as the extent and site of any brain damage.

Personality also has its part to play in a child's learning pattern. Whether a child is introverted or extroverted, determined or gives in easily, creative or not, adaptable or rigid, self-motivated or otherwise, impetuous or considered, such qualities will all affect the way in which she approaches learning. Her personality will have an effect on all aspects of the child's development, and the encouragement of positive personality traits likely to help her to reach maximum potential is as important as physical exercise and intellectual stimulation.

Because of the mobility problems experienced by children who have cerebral palsy it is highly likely that the development of their understanding can be greatly assisted if parents and professionals ensure that they receive normal environmental stimuli, including an emphasis on movement.

Some children with CP do appear to have learning difficulties but this is not necessarily related to the degree of physical disability. Having a learning difficulty does not take away your personality and individuality. Parents may fear this because of the common attitude in society that those who have learning difficulties are less whole than those who do not. There is no optimum level of knowledge and understanding. Every individual, disabled or not, will be different in how and what they know and perceive. I have met many people who have been labelled as having learning difficulties who have a perception of the world and of themselves which I admire and aspire to. I have met many people without learning difficulties whom I do not.

## Can cerebral palsy get worse as the child gets older?

A part of the brain has been irreparably damaged but the damage will not get any worse unless the child suffers further damage due to a separate incident. It is possible in many instances for children who have cerebral palsy to gain increasingly greater control over their movement. This may be due to treatment, determination on the part of the child, partial recovery of the brain or just something inexplicable. In some cases the child will appear to recover totally. Total recovery is only likely to happen where the symptoms are not too severe and will take place very early on in the child's life, usually in the first year. A study done by Nelson and Ellenberg in 1982 showed that only 111 of 229 children who were suspected to have cerebral palsy under the age of one went on to develop cerebral palsy by the age of 7. There are a number of theories as to why this happens. The most commonly held theory is that where damage is not too severe the still developing brain can take compensatory measures or, more simply, another part of the brain takes over the function of the damaged area. The damage is still present in the brain but the child's ability to function is restored.

It is also possible for a child to seem to have less control over his movement as time goes on. This is likely to be due to the fact that the effect of the brain damage becomes more apparent as the child get older rather than to any deterioration in the child's condition. Very rarely cysts on the brain may cause excessive fluid to build up on the brain (hydrocephalus), the pressure of which can cause brain damage. This condition can be relieved by medical treatment or an operation.

## Is the child only likely to have difficulties with movement?

This will depend on the extent to which the child's brain has been damaged and which areas of her brain are affected. She may also have difficulty seeing, hearing and speaking. She may be able to see and hear but unable to make sense of what she is seeing and hearing. She may have fits of epilepsy which can be either severe or mild. Some children with cerebral palsy have difficulty organising information although they are of normal intelligence. Other children may appear to be intellectually impaired.

Medical research is continually increasing the understanding of the causes and classifications of cerebral palsy, allowing preventative measures to be improved. The ability of doctors to isolate the particular problems a child may have in muscle and bone development is constantly improving. This enables the doctor to suggest treatment methods designed to counter the effects which the brain damage is having on muscle development and potential bone deformity. There is still a great deal about the functioning of the brain which is not understood.

On the other hand, isolated concentration on scientific enquiry and medical classification can serve as a distraction from the social and environmental needs of the child who has cerebral palsy. While we concentrate on causes and classifications our attention is diverted from the injustice and inequality in the social world within which the child with cerebral palsy lives and the non-medical measures which could be taken to enable her to enjoy a full life. This is discussed further in Chapter 1.

## Statistics on incidence and prevalence

*Incidence* is the number of new cases occurring during a certain time period in a particular population considered to be at risk – for example, the number of cases per 1000 premature births.

*Prevalence* is the number of cases occurring during a certain time period in an overall population for example, the number of cases per 1000 live births.

Despite improved obstetric care it has been noted that there was no significant change in the prevalence of cerebral palsy among children born in the North of England between 1960 and 1976. The range of severity has not been noted to change over time either. It has been suggested that this could be due to the fact that more sophisticated methods of resuscitation are now leading to the survival of children who, 10 years ago, would have died at the same time as enabling others, who would have just survived 10 years ago with severe disability, to now present with more mild disabilities as treatment techniques continue to improve.

The total prevalence of cerebral palsy is generally reckoned to be 2 per 1000 live births (0.2 per cent). However, it has been suggested that this figure is artificially low because of the late diagnosis of many cases and a number of mild cases that go undiagnosed. Taking this into account the figure could be as high as 5 per 1000 live births (0.5 per cent).

A review of prevalence studies undertaken in the 1980s revealed prevalence rates varying from 1 to 5.8 per 1000 live births with the higher figures occurring in groups of children tested over the age of 5. It has also been noted that the prevalence rises in times of epidemics of 'flu and where environmental factors such as a high incidence of malnutrition – due to poverty for example – prevail. In almost all studies, approximately 10 per cent of cases are thought to be of postnatal origin.

In 1967 Mcdonald undertook a study which established that 7.9 per cent of singleton low-birthweight survivors and 3.1 per cent of multiple low-birthweight survivors (i.e. twins, triplets or more) were diagnosed as having cerebral palsy. Of these, 81 per cent had spastic diplegia, 4 per cent had choreoathetosis, 4 per cent had spastic quadriplegia, 3 per cent had spastic hemiplegia and 8 per cent had other syndromes.

With severe asphyxia in infants born at term (after a pregnancy of 37 weeks or more), it is generally found that severe spastic quadriplegia is the most common result with a small number of children presenting with athetosis. Asphyxia in pre-term infants is more likely to result in spastic diplegia and minimal other handicap.

Contrary to earlier popular belief, it has been found that asphyxia at birth is not a major cause of cerebral palsy. Only 10 per cent of cases are known to have this cause, and in many of the other cases the damage will either have occurred earlier or will be sustained some time after the baby has been born.

A New York study found that 73.4 per cent of children with cerebral palsy had a spastic form of the condition, 12.5 per cent were ataxic, 7 per cent were mixed, 3 per cent had rigidity, 1 per cent were athetoid and 0.5 per cent had tremors. This study also found that 47 per cent had quadriplegia, 46 per cent had hemiplegia and 5 per cent paraplegia.

Cerebral palsy is a varied condition. The rest of this book will hopefully equip you with the information you need to make decisions to help ensure that your child gets maximum opportunity to enjoy a full life, whatever his condition.

# 1

# Should therapy and treatment be your first priority?

'A disabled child has the right to enjoy a full and decent life, in conditions which ensure dignity, promote self-reliance, and facilitate the child's active participation in the community.'
(UN Convention on the Rights of the Child, 1989)

The type and amount of therapy and treatment you are offered will vary enormously depending on the area you are living in. You have the choice to say 'yes' or 'no' to what you are offered and to seek alternative forms of support from other areas and the private sector (although the latter almost always costs money and this may pose problems).

Before I suggest ways in which you can help your child using various medical and therapeutic techniques I would like you to consider your child's needs in relation to the world he is going to grow up in. This is probably going to affect his ability to develop and grow just as much, and with equally far-reaching implications, as the amount of physiotherapy and other therapy he receives.

Begin by considering the following statements and mark whether you agree, strongly agree, disagree or strongly disagree.

When you have marked the statements, think about why you marked them as you did. Are you feeling that your child must become as near 'normal' as possible? Do you feel that this is the only way he can live a fulfilled life? Do you feel that there is something wrong with your child? Have you considered his social and friendship needs as well as his need to perform everyday activities such as walking and talking? Do you feel that he will only have a full social life if he walks and talks? Are you concerned that he should get 'better'? Do you

I want my child to enjoy life
I want my child to have lots of friends
I want my child to be able to make choices
I want my child to go to an ordinary school
I want my child to walk
I want my child to talk
I want my child to be able to use her hands
I want my child to see
I want my child to hear
I want my child to lead a normal life
I want my child to be intelligent
If my child does not learn to walk she will not be a happy
    person
If my child does not learn to walk I will not be a happy
    person
People with disabilities must try to fit in with society
Society should be changed so that disabled people's needs
    can be met more easily
There is nothing a disabled person cannot do with the
    right support

feel that the whole thing is too big for you to handle? Would
you prefer to entrust your child's development to 'professionals'? Do you distrust the professionals and feel that you
should go all out to find a better way to help your child? Do
you feel that therapy and treatment is a waste of time and that
it is more important to enable your child to be accepted for who
he is as he is? Are you afraid that your child will not live up to
your expectations? Are you afraid that you will not be able to
live up to your own expectations as carer of your child?

Many of these questions could be asked of the parent of a
non-disabled child. The difference is that your situation is less
predictable with a few extra problems tagged on. A lot of
expectations tend to get placed on disabled people in order that
they will fit in better to a non-disabled world. We are all
conditioned to expect certain behaviour and abilities from our
children and our expectations are based on our knowledge of
what is considered 'normal' in the social circle and environment we live in. If our children are not able to fulfil our
expectations not only are we likely to panic but so are those
around us. How well your child is able to integrate into society
and live a full life within it is likely to be heavily influenced by

your attitude towards her in her early years of life. Your attitude will influence the attitudes of others she comes into contact with. These attitudes will in turn affect her confidence and ability to take her place in the world.

## The historical context

Disability has been seen differently at various points in history. The Greeks used to kill children who were born disabled as they were regarded either as economic burdens who served no useful purpose or as retribution from the gods. In the 18th century in Britain 'cripples' were considered to be lower class citizens along with beggars, the unemployed and those who had fallen from grace through vice.

In the late 18th century institutions started to spring up to which people with disabilities could be removed. These were not places of care and treatment but places where those considered a burden and an embarrassment could be kept away from ordinary life where their bodily needs would be met without disruption to society.

As recently as 50–100 years ago, compulsory sterilisation of people considered to be mentally handicapped was taking place in the USA on the theory that it was necessary to reduce the number of 'mental defects' being produced in society.

In the 18th century there was a fairly successful move in the deaf community to promote communication by signing. However, under the influence of a school of thought inspired by Charles Darwin, which held that 'defectives' were unnatural and every measure should be taken to eradicate disability, attempts were made to ban signing and to stop deaf people from marrying each other in case it led to the human race becoming deaf. This suppression is still having its effect today with strong debate still carrying on between those professionals who support signing and those who feel that deaf people must learn to speak in order to fit into society. This is even though there is strong evidence that children who are not allowed to sign are less likely to achieve academically, and are more vulnerable to child abuse, because they have had their means of early communication taken away from them. There are many deaf people today who can remember having their hands tied behind their backs in school in an attempt to force them to communicate orally.

## The position of people with disabilities today

A more humane approach has recently developed (alongside advances in technology) which involves every attempt being made to render the child as near to non-disabled as possible with the use of drugs, surgery and therapy. The emphasis remains on creating as little obvious sign of disability in public as possible.

An increasing number of people with disabilities are becoming involved in the disability rights movement and finding ways to make their voices heard. The main focus of the movement is to argue for equal rights for those who have disabilities. The movement does not necessarily object to treatment and therapy but the emphasis is on persuading the local community and society at large that people with disabilities can be accommodated and make a positive contribution as they are.

There are different ways in which we can look at disability. Religious leaders in history have justified gross acts of inhumanity towards people with disabilities. I am not suggesting that religion is wrong, only that it has been misused by people in positions of power to justify the segregation and mistreatment of a section of society who were misunderstood and undervalued.

The medical view of disability is the most common viewpoint held today. The main thrust of this view is that people with disabilities should be 'treated', 'changed', 'improved' and made more 'normal'. The medical view looks at the problems which disabled children are seen to have and apply therapeutic, medical and special teaching techniques in order that they will be better able to fit into the world as it stands.

The disability movement views the needs of children who have disabilities in terms of the social world they live in. They look around at the environment and suggest changes which could be made to it to better enable them to enjoy full and active lives.

We don't have to look far before we come up against barriers to progress: ill-equipped mainstream schools and work places, lack of adequate training for teachers and employers, funding geared towards treatments rather than adaptations in the environment, ignorance and fear on the part of the majority of the population which drives carers of children with disabilities indoors to hide their children from cruel stares and remarks. There is no forum in which people with disabilities can be publicly heard. The main focus of the disability rights movement is to ensure that people with disabilities have as much of a say in the running of society as any other citizen. Children with disabilities rely on those who care for them to be their advocates and we need to do all we can to ensure that they get access to equal opportunities.

There are numerous organisations which have been set up to provide information and practical help for people who have disabilities. Most of these organisations are run for people with disabilities rather than by them. Some make every effort to get people with disabilities onto the Committee of Management but, in the main, organisations which set out to improve the quality of life for the disabled are organised and controlled by non-disabled people.

## Considerations for parents and carers

While you are considering what steps to take to help your child it is always worth asking the question: 'For whose benefit?' I'm not suggesting that children with cerebral palsy should not receive treatment or that they should not be given every opportunity to develop educationally. All children need assistance to develop and flourish and a child with disabilities is no exception. They may even require some extra input to enable them to develop to their own satisfaction. I am, however, asking you to consider which steps are necessary for your child's well-being and which might arguably be for the convenience of you, your family, the therapists and other specialists you will meet and the preservation of a status quo in society at large.

The problems begin with the lack of day to day contact between disabled and non-disabled people. Research has shown that up to 88 per cent of non-disabled people are not in regular contact with a person who has a physical disability. To answer the question of why there is such lack of contact we need to examine the opportunity for contact. For many children this begins as soon as they are recognised as having a visible disability. Parents may react in a number of ways but two common reactions are:

- A desire to protect your child from physical and emotional harm
- Embarrassment about your child's disability.

Another factor which may influence the early segregation of children comes from medical and educational establishments. A significant amount of the child's time can be taken up in visits to specialists, hospital admissions, medical and psychological assessments, physiotherapy and administration of drugs. A host of well meaning interventions can combine to take up almost the whole of a child's waking existence. This can lead to isolation, not only of the child, but of the carer as well. Also, the scene is set in which the child is perceived as 'different', first and foremost, with the emphasis being on her child having to work towards eliminating this difference. Yet this very aim is sometimes contradicted by the unusual environment which the treatment situation often constructs for children who have disabilities. Therapy should *complement* normal life, not replace it.

Can you imagine how you yourself could have developed into a normal adult if your main stimulation as a child was to be pushed and pulled about constantly and against your will, sometimes painfully and often causing discomfort? To add to this, if anyone remembered to let you play it was only in a structured and orderly way and never enabling you the opportunity of spontaneous expression. The final insult being that you seemed to spend half your life being carted from one sterile environment to another where men and women in white coats would peer at you without actually noticing that you had any feelings or even that you knew that they were there. They would proceed to talk over your head, not about you but about bits of your body and whether you had a mind, and all the while you were unable to express the frustration and confusion you felt at the undignified treatment.

As the child gets older the situation worsens rather than improves. It is very difficult for children who have any but the mildest of disabilities to gain automatic access to integrated educational opportunities. It is even more difficult for adults to gain access to properly paid employment. This is not necessarily because the disabled person is not able to undertake the education or employment but more often because there is a lack of basic amenities to enable them to participate equally. Such amenities include accessible buildings, appropriate equipment and properly trained assistants to help in the classroom or workplace.

It is highly likely that your child will need a therapeutic exercise programme but it is important to remember that the exercises should be slotted into a normal everyday life which will enable your child to lead a full, happy and active existence. Never forget the place of unstructured play, relaxation, and the right to make choices.

Making choices is an essential part of learning as we grow up. Not all choices made by small children are appropriate, however, and a child with disabilities requires discipline in her life just as a non-disabled child does. It should be appreciated, though, that refusal to acknowledge a child's protests against a plainly uncomfortable experience, which is being administered by the adult to whom she must turn for a role model, may lead that child to lose a very important developmental guide.

As a carer of a disabled child you may be asked to carry out appropriate measures in the home to enable your child's development. Some of the advice will be excellent and appropriate to your individual child's needs. Other advice may not be. Only you, knowing the child so well, can decide which activities work and which need changing or throwing out. Professionals can have a way of making you feel that failure to follow their precise instructions will have catastrophic effects. It should be remembered that parents, therapists, doctors and educators are all professionals who should be working together in real partnership for the benefit of the child. The professional offering you advice will probably have a wide experience of similar situations but we are all capable of making mistakes and misinterpreting situations. It is the service of your child's emotional, physical and intellectual needs which is paramount.

A professional who is willing to listen to your views, accept your preferences and amend his advice accordingly is more likely to be able to support you in providing your child with beneficial treatment and training. Professionals who constantly quote textbooks and methods tested by experimental design may lack the ability to recognise the truly unique person which every child is.

A positive attitude towards a child is essential. Children with disabilities (like any children) need praise and encouragement, and to be respected for who they are, not who you might be trying to make them be.

You may decide to opt for private therapy or training. For

economic reasons you may not have this choice. If you can and do choose this route remember that you are still the carer and you still control the situation for the benefit of your child.

As your child gets older the pressure to conform to society's convenience increases. Special schools and special units in mainstream schools are still a preferred option in many local authorities especially if your child is considered to have a learning difficulty and it seems to affect his understanding.

Arguments against integrated education include: lack of financial resources, lack of trained staff, disruption of 'normal' teaching and inaccessibility of buildings.

During my research I discussed integration with those working in special schools and was surprised to find that there was significant support for integration 'if only the resources were available'! It might be appropriate to consider where existing resources, scarce as they are, are being channelled. A great deal of the existing resources are channelled into the research and development of medical 'solutions' rather than environmental adaptations to improve the disabled person's opportunity to participate.

Chapter 7 will examine the arguments which have been put for and against special and segregated education. The point I want to make here is that you need to be sure of your reasons for the choice you make about your child's education. If you choose to have him educated in a special school, is it because you are certain that the special environment really offers your child the best hope of an independent future? Or is it because you have been pressured by a Local Authority whose resources are currently organised with a non-disabled orientation?

Finally, the biggest hurdle many people with disabilities face is what happens after the age of 19? Many carers have said to me that this is their biggest worry. At the age of 19 the support which might have been offered within school melts away and the teenager is suddenly catapulted from a protected, often segregated, environment into an adult world which is hostile to his needs. Furthermore it is unlikely that even medical resources will be channelled towards the disabled adult, these being reserved mainly for the young. This issue and the options available are further addressed in Chapter 8.

# 2

# The early stages

## Recognising and dealing with problems

### Recognising the symptoms

If your child was born prematurely, had a trauma at birth or an accident after birth, you will probably have been made aware of the possibility that she could have brain damage. For many people, however, the realisation that there is something wrong comes very slowly.

The following signs might occur which cause concern for carers.

**1–3 months (and older):**
- Does not kick;
- Seems stiff or unduly floppy;
- Asymmetrical – for example, more active on one side than the other;
- Takes a long time to feed, poor sucking reflex;
- Does not smile by 8–10 weeks;
- Eyes do not meet mother's;
- Does not follow object held 6 inches away and moved horizontally;

**3–6 months (and older):**
- Still unable to hold up head;
- Does not put hand in mouth;
- Limbs seem very stiff (as if the muscle were always tight);
- Limbs very floppy;
- Head thrown back;
- Feet turning out;
- Legs crossing in scissor action;
- Feet pointed at toes rather than flat;
- Tendency to curl up in a foetal position;
- Tendency to throw arms and body backwards;
- Eyes rolling backwards or sideways;

- Not turning to sound;
- Extra sensitivity to touch demonstrated by excessive crying on physical contact;
- Does not seem to recognise familiar people;
- Is not cooing, gurgling or, later, babbling;
- Does not reach for objects;
- Does not roll over from front to side;
- Dislikes being on stomach. Unable to lift head in this position

Many of the signs of cerebral palsy are actually reflexes and responses which are naturally present in a newborn baby but which usually disappear after a few weeks. This makes it very difficult to diagnose CP in the early days of life. It is only as those early reflexes and motor patterns persist past the appropriate age that cause for concern becomes apparent.

Table 2 shows a brief outline of development progress with average ages given. If your child is not progressing exactly as outlined in this chart there is no automatic need for concern; it is only a guide. However, it is likely that a child who has cerebral palsy (unless very mildly affected) will show significant difference in his development.

## Getting a diagnosis

My own research suggests that in 57 per cent of cases, official diagnosis took place six months or more after problems had been picked up by parents. In 29 per cent of cases it took in excess of a year for a diagnosis to be provided. While it is understandable that doctors may be unwilling to diagnose straight away given the incidence of recovery in the early months, I believe that 12 months plus is an unacceptable time lag and parents are well justified in demanding an honest appraisal of their child's condition if one has not been offered by the age of 12 months. It is usually appropriate for a child to begin being assessed and given exercises by a physiotherapist before a definite diagnosis can be made.

Many parents have reported that they felt the consultant had knowledge of a diagnosis well before they were told. It is extremely helpful if carers can be told as early as possible as it has been suggested on numerous occasions that early therapeutic intervention can help to limit the damaging effects of cerebral palsy.

**Table 2** Brief outline of average child development. Based on the work of Sheridan (1975), Levitt (1978) and others

| Age | Gross motor (body movements) | Vision and fine motor (hand/eye co-ordination) | Hearing and speech | Social, emotional self-care |
|---|---|---|---|---|
| 1–3 months | – Head flops if sat up<br>– Jerky kicks when on back<br>– Becomes less likely to curl up when handled | – Watches mother's face<br>– Turns to light<br>– Thumb rests in palm<br>– Has automatic grasp but can't let go | – Startles to loud noise<br>– Stills to familiar gentle sounds<br>– Cries when hungry or if uncomfortable | – Sleeps frequently<br>– Social smile by 8 weeks<br>– Appears alert<br>– Sucks well |
| 3–6 months | – Holds head up independently<br>– Leans on forearms and raises head<br>– Can roll from front to side<br>– Can sit up with support | – Gazes around. Visually alert<br>– Becomes able to reach out and touch object being looked at<br>– Takes interest in object in hand | – Coos, gurgles and (by 6 months) babbles<br>– Turns to sound<br>– Communicates by moving (e.g. begins to raise arm to indicate wish to be picked up) | – Recognises people<br>– Can show pleasure and excitement<br>– Lips, tongue and swallowing become active. Capable of dealing with soft food<br>– Hands can be placed on bottle |
| 6–9 months | – Can roll from back to stomach<br>– Can sit alone<br>– Pats a mirror image<br>– Goes up on all fours | – Watches dropped object but forgets it when can no longer see it<br>– Can pass objects from one hand to another<br>– Mouths objects | – Chuckles, laughs, squeals and screams<br>– Turns quickly to mother's voice<br>– Listens attentively<br>– Practises sounds | – Recognises tone of voice<br>– Responds differently to strangers<br>– Holds bottle or cup and drinks |

| Age | Gross motor (body movements) | Vision and fine motor (hand/eye co-ordination) | Hearing and speech | Social, emotional self-care |
|---|---|---|---|---|
| 9–12 months | – Rolls to change positions, lying, sitting etc.<br>– Crawls<br>– Stands supported<br>– Walks holding on or alone at 12 months | – Takes object out of container<br>– Quick to visually scan environment and select desired object<br>– Uses fingers in isolation from each other<br>– Prods, pokes and later points with index finger | – Babbles using purposeful sounds<br>– Begins to understand words, gestures. Knows name, 'no' and may say some understandable words. Understands more than says<br>– Waves 'bye bye' | – Reacts to encouragement<br>– Shows many emotions<br>– Plays peek-a-boo and searches for hidden objects<br>– Offers toy to others<br>– Wary of strangers<br>– Holds spoon and may take to mouth but overturns it. Messy feeder. Drinks alone if guided. Chews<br>– Imitates others |
| 12–18 months | – Walking alone, after walking with one hand held<br>– May begin stiff running<br>– Kneels unaided<br>– Squats at play<br>– Stands and stoops to pick up toy | – Can pick up small crumbs<br>– Can build 2/3 block tower once shown how<br>– Scribbles with crude grasp<br>– Points to pictures and enjoys books<br>– Mouthing objects less | – Attends to words being spoken. Uses about 6–20 words.<br>– Echoes some words<br>– Obeys simple instructions<br>– Points to body parts<br>– Enjoys nursery jingles<br>– Names of people and things understood | – Picks up cup/spoon and takes to mouth<br>– Puts out arms and legs for dressing<br>– Restless to indicate toilet need<br>– Plays alone but near others<br>– Objects put in and out of containers |
| 18 months to 2 years | – Runs less stiffly<br>– Walks up stairs holding on<br>– Throws ball with direction<br>– Walks backwards pulling toy by string | – Removes wrapping from sweets<br>– Circular scribbles and dots<br>– Turns single pages, book right way up | – Uses about 50 words<br>– Refers to self by name. Puts two or more words together<br>– Joins in nursery rhymes | – Indicates toilet needs<br>– Able to undress a little<br>– Independent feeding<br>– Make-believe play<br>– Does not realise dangers |

| Age | | | | |
|---|---|---|---|---|
| 2–2½ years | – Climbs easy apparatus<br>– Kicks large ball<br>– Jumps with two feet together<br>– May be able to tricycle a little | – Builds tower of 6–8 blocks<br>– Quick recognition of pictures in book<br>– Paints dots, strokes<br>– May hold crayon with first two fingers and thumb | – 200 or more words<br>– Questions and pronouns<br>– Enjoys simple stories<br>– Says some rhymes<br>– Names some body parts<br>– Follows directions, e.g. up, down etc. | – Eats skilfully with spoon. May use fork<br>– Puts on hat and shoes<br>– Active, restless and rebellious. Tantrums<br>– May join in make-believe play with others<br>– Cannot understand sharing |
| 2½–3 years | – Goes up stairs with alternative feet<br>– Agile climbing<br>– Avoids obstacles<br>– Can run or walk on tiptoe | – Imitates finger play<br>– Can copy a cross and draw body with head and one other part of body<br>– Cuts with scissors<br>– Paints at easel | – Listens to story attentively<br>– Others can understand what he is saying<br>– Often asks for favourite story<br>– Counts without knowing meaning of quantity | – Washes hands but needs help drying<br>– Takes off and puts on clothes except buttons<br>– Likes to help adult<br>– Understands sharing<br>– Left and right confused in dressing |
| 3–4 years | – Climbs ladders and trees<br>– Stands on one leg for 5 seconds<br>– Hops on same leg<br>– Throws and catches ball | – Draws a body with head, trunk, legs, arms, fingers<br>– Matches about four colours<br>– Can thread beads | – Speech grammar correct<br>– Can describe recent events<br>– Jokes, tells long stories and fantasises<br>– Counts to 20 | – Can wash and dry hands<br>– Dresses with buttoning but not laces<br>– Takes turns<br>– Appreciates past, present and future<br>– Protective to others |
| 4–5 years | – Can dance, skip, hop on either leg<br>– Can walk on narrow line | – Copies square, letters<br>– Can draw person and house with detail<br>– Counts fingers<br>– Matches and names colours | – Fluent speech<br>– Acts out stories<br>– Enjoys jokes | – Knife and fork used<br>– Undresses and dresses<br>– Relates to friends |

Doctors may find the emotional experience of telling a parent that their child has a disability extremely distressing. Added to this their past experience in dealing with severe disability and feelings of frustration when faced with a disabling condition they know they cannot cure may lead to a tendency on the part of doctors to take a negative stand in regard to the future of a child with cerebral palsy. Counselling skills are not taught to doctors in any depth and nearly all of their training is geared towards cure through the use of surgery and drugs. This leaves the odds fairly stacked against a positive relationship developing between the carers, who are likely to be highly motivated to do all they can to help their child, and the consultant whose training leaves him in a relatively helpless situation when faced with caring parents and a child whom he may feel unable to treat.

Reading through comments made by other carers I was overwhelmed by the almost unanimous opinion that the consultant was/is unhelpful and unnecessarily negative. In contrast, physiotherapists were seen as supportive and helpful. In many cases the physiotherapist is reported to offer the first positive support carers receive from professionals involved in the care of their child.

This enormous body of opinion from clients suggests that the medical profession might benefit from a revaluation of the current approach to children with disabilities and their carers.

Fear of overestimating a child's abilities and consequent disappointment to carers, possibly coupled with their own uncertainty regarding a child's future, can lead doctors to play down a child's potential.

I do not want to give the impression that the medical profession is entirely peopled by uncaring and insensitive beings. My first consultant was keenly interested in my opinion and willing to keep a completely open mind on Danny's prognosis. They do exist! Doctors are themselves let down by the emphasis on correction and cure and lack of concern with support and interactive dialogue with patients in their training.

## Parents' first reactions and support in the early days

There are a variety of immediate reactions which a family might have when they realise their child has a permanent disability. How they feel about it will be affected by many influences such as: what personal experience they have of disability, how they are told, what attitudes they already have about disability, whether they had considered the possibility before of having a child who is disabled.

It is commonly believed amongst medical professionals that parents go through a process of grieving which is very similar to the reaction to be expected at the death of a child. This process progresses from shock to anger, guilt, grief and eventually, what is termed acceptance. Many books and professionals stress the importance of 'coming to terms with a child's disability'. This may well be a true reflection of the reactions of some parents. However, it may not need to be this way. Research carried out by Chris Goodey between 1987 and 1989 revealed that many parents felt that their feelings were influenced by the attitudes of doctors and other health professionals who talked to them about their children after diagnosis. Unfortunately these attitudes were often negative. 'I'm afraid your child is disabled.' 'I'm sorry to have to tell you but. . . .' Chris Goodey gives a number of examples of cases where parents feel that they were prepared for what happened and were willing to welcome their children but where the professionals involved were distressed and uncomfortable, even to the point of crying or being unable to look at the parents when discussing the situation with them. This kind of reaction from professional people who we hope have our best interests at heart can only at best produce confusion and at worst actually create the experience of grief for the parents.

There is no logical reason for feeling badly towards or about a young child. There may be plenty of reason to feel unhappy about lack of information, money, advice and practical support, all of which are commonly a problem for families who have a member who is disabled. The only reason anyone would harbour negative thoughts about children with disabilities is when someone in authority, or a body of opinion, advises that this is the natural thing to do.

Parents of a disabled child may be thrust into a situation they probably did not expect, which is generally perceived in negative terms and feared with dread by many prospective parents and medical professionals and about which there may be very little information available. However, many parents report very positive feelings towards and involvement with their child.

Negative attitudes and beliefs ae not likely to change overnight. The best action parents can probably take is to make contact with self-help support groups as early as possible so that they can share information and experiences with others in a similar situation. If your health visitor doesn't know of any in your area Scope or the cerebral palsy helpline may know of them.

I have heard it suggested in some professional circles that parents should be left to get to know their child for a few months before the professionals come into the home offering support and developmental advice. While respect for the privacy of the family is to be applauded this cannot become a standard approach. Each family is unique in its needs and interpersonal relationships. Given the chance, many families will know what they need most and it may be that the professional involved at the beginning has a role in enabling the family to establish priorities.

The first point of contact is likely to be with the doctor who diagnoses your child. The second point of contact is likely to be the health visitor. In a very few areas a special needs health visitor will be available whose responsibility it is to link the hospital input with the community as well as offering carers and children general support in early health care. The family may need help with getting a clearer understanding of their new situation. I refrain from using their terms 'learning to cope with' or 'coming to terms with' because, if handled properly, these negative images of disability can be avoided in the very early stages. Referral to counselling for the family may be appropriate, and is discussed in more detail in Chapter 3.

One of the early difficulties will be uncertainty around a child's prognosis (likely outcome as he grows up). There have been a number of studies designed to establish whether outcomes can be predicted. It has been found that the specific type of cerebral palsy may be an important factor in independent living. However, there are numbers of adults with severe quadriplegia (where medical prognosis is not good) who have fine jobs and good standing in the local community. It has also been found that some children who have sustained minimal damage become severely disabled while others who appear to have sustained severe damage are only slightly affected in motor ability. According to one study, the employment outlook was best for those who had spastic paralysis and who had attended regular school. However, it is important to recognise that employment opportunity and other outcomes are as dependent on the construction of the environment as on the development of the individual. I would suggest that these studies are showing which groups are most likely to be able to 'fit into' the non-disabled world rather than any indicator of ability and future prospects given the right community support and opportunity.

In 1981, Soboloff followed up 248 adults who had cerebral palsy who were between the ages of 20 and 50. He found that 48 per cent were self-sufficient community walkers; 30 per cent had part-time care and used a wheelchair except for household walking; 22 per cent were having total care and considered to be helpless; 31 per cent were in full-time employment (the majority of these people had spastic diplegia or hemiplegia); about one-third were housebound or institutionalised; 8 per cent had married, and 15 of the original 248 had died.

In my own study the most popular question parents asked when their children were diagnosed was, 'What will her prospects be?' This was followed in order by, 'Will she walk?' 'What caused it?' 'Can she be cured?' 'How severe is it?' 'Will she be mentally handicapped?' 'Will she talk?' 'What treatment is available?' 'How can I help her?' 'What is cerebral palsy?' and 'Will future children be the same?'

These are all difficult questions to answer however experienced the consultant. Quoting statistics on outcomes will not provide a formula for your child's development. So much in any child's life depends on factors unique to that child's situation. The family can help its own children enormously by having a positive attitude towards them and helping them to grow and develop. The medical or child development team can provide back up to families. If you do not feel that you are getting enough support you could try contacting the local Scope social worker or your local social services department to voice your concerns regarding the support you are receiving.

There can be so much benefit to the family who is listened to, given time, given honest answers to their questions, allowed the opportunity to air their fears and express their emotions and then fully supported both emotionally and practically to welcome their child who has disabilities into the family as an equal member with a positive contribution to make.

## Getting an early start to a treatment programme

This is a difficult issue. Many parents and carers feel that they have a desperate race against time to do all they can to moderate the effect of their child's brain damage. Others need considerable time to get used to the unexpected situation before contemplating action. Many activists in the disability movement (most of whom have disabilities) believe it is wrong to thrust the young child into programmes of treatment which they see as invasive, cruel and of dubious value.

Some medical studies have suggested that treatment programmes based on exercises have not been proved to be effective but these studies usually accompany research designed to show the effectiveness of the medical interventions such as surgery and drugs. Other studies suggest that the effects of drugs and surgery can be as detrimental as they are likely to be beneficial. The truth of the matter is that no profession has yet come up with the magical intervention which can be guaranteed to help a child to maximise her potential.

What you can be offered by the Health Service will be determined by a number of factors: the resources (money, staff and equipment) available in your area, the attitudes and beliefs of those who provide the service, whether particular methods are preferred by your local service, the type of service delivery, the relationship between your health authority and other sorts of support which might be locally available (such as special interest groups, local branches of Scope etc.)

There are also a number of options available in a private market, which may or may not be beneficial to your child and may or may not be out of reach of your pocket.

## Normal life comes first

Giving your child every opportunity to have a normal life comes before any consideration of special and/or unusual treatments and training programmes designed to support your child's development. Our earliest learning is not achieved by our carers alone inputting information into us. It is now a well established fact that children, from a very early age, often initiate interaction between themselves and their carers. For example, there have been studies carried out which demonstrated mothers 'teaching' their very small babies to develop early language by copying their child's first babbling. The baby says 'aah ba ga' and the mother responds with 'aahoa ba ba ba ga ga ga'. Without realising it we are being led by our children into extending their early vocabulary. This process of interaction is augmented by a fairly predictable pattern which most children develop. In their early days this consists mainly of crying followed by feeding followed by sleeping. Gradually the child will spend longer and longer awake and quietly (or loudly in some cases!) attending to the world around him. Later he begins to explore with first his eyes, then his hands. As the child's natural curiosity unfolds, his mobility will increase. Along with this increased mobility comes further opportunity to learn about the small environment in which he lives simply through exploration. By the age of 6 months a child is likely to have mastered rolling over to get closer to a desired object and possibly sitting to gain an alternative perspective. By one year, children have developed some means of travelling across small distances to reach a desired object and will be pulling themselves up to get at objects they can't reach from a lying position. By 18 months most children have mastered the art of walking and, once this is achieved, their vocabulary often makes dramatic progress.

All of this takes place without the need for conscious effort on the part of the carer to enable the process. Even if we are preoccupied with other things the child will find a way to discover the world and learn by experience and experiment. A child who has cerebral palsy is disadvantaged from the earliest point of this natural development process, starting with the early emotional life.

Children with cerebral palsy may have difficulty in giving their parents the cues that normally facilitate development in a reciprocal way. If a child is unable to put out the communication which sparks off the necessary adult response, her development could be impeded. We can help to reinstate this process with a little thought and appropriate advice. The local educational psychologist, peripatetic teacher or speech and language therapist may be able to offer some advice on play and ways of being with our children. If you have older children, reminding yourself of the way you interacted with them may help. I found it well worth while to invest in a couple of books on child development and play (which were not aimed at children with disabilities) to remind myself of the kind of play activity which might be appropriate for Danny's age group (see the further reading section for guidance on this).

Lots of stimulation from very early on will aid your child's natural development. This doesn't necessarily mean that you have to be attending to your child every second of the day but it does mean that you will need to provide opportunities. For example, if you are leaving your child to play on her own while you do housework or attend the needs of another child, surround your child with stimulating toys which move, produce sounds and/or have bright reflective colours. The sound and bright colours are particularly important if your child is suspected to have difficulties with hearing and vision.

Playing music to small children is also very stimulating. Classical music can be particularly entertaining because it has a complexity which will keep a child's attention longer than pop music or even nursery rhymes. Nursery rhymes are excellent for helping a child to gain a sense of rhythm and producing action through rhythm.

Start reading stories to your child as early as possible. Show him pictures, shapes and puzzles and, most importantly, talk to him.

A running commentary on what you are doing will help your child to develop understanding, keep her amused and get her involved in family life.

## Medical considerations

### Vaccination

Every child is likely to go through the usual round of childhood illnesses such as chicken pox, tummy upsets and the common cold. Previously common illnesses, such as measles, mumps and whooping cough, can be vaccinated against but some parents do not believe in vaccination. Children with cerebral palsy may appear to react more strongly than other children when they catch a commonplace illness. Commonplace illnesses can increase spasm, further inhibit control over movement and set back development – especially if during the illness exercise programmes and other routines need to stop.

If your child is normally on an exercise programme which cannot be carried out due to illness, he will be likely to show signs of temporary deterioration in muscle control as well as the common symptoms associated with the illness. For this reason alone it is worth seriously considering having your child vaccinated against common complaints where a vaccination is available. It may be well worth your while to ensure that your child does not get held up by common illnesses any more than is necessary.

Some parents are concerned about dangerous side-effects from certain vaccinations. The whooping cough vaccination has particularly been highlighted as having potential dangers. These days even the whooping cough vaccination is recommended for virtually all children who have brain damage.

## Unusual sleep and attention patterns

I was frustrated to find that my experience of a sleepless, unhappy baby was not uncommon. Furthermore, I discovered that his constant constipation was also experienced by a lot of children who have cerebral palsy. If someone had told me that these problems were associated with CP, and not due to my inadequate mothering, I might have cottoned on to remedial action a great deal sooner.

If your child is stiff it is quite likely that she will get uncomfortable at night and wake more frequently than a baby who does not have disabilities. On the other hand, a floppy child or one who is taking barbiturates to control fits may seem lethargic and appear to be an overly 'good' baby. I have spoken to mothers who have been concerned about providing their baby with stimulation and play opportunities but have had difficulty waking their child up, and keeping her awake.

Many parents of children with CP notice that they cry a lot more than their siblings, or other children they have known. Other parents express concern that their baby just 'lies there' demonstrating no emotion. If a child is suffering discomfort as a result of his disability it is no surprise that he expresses this in the only way a small child is able – by giving out distress signals through crying. If your child is extremely quiet and is also being administered drugs it may be that the side-effects of the drugs are actually having a sedative effect which may impede his natural development process – although this is not necessarily always the case.

Whether your child cries a lot or is abnormally quiet the natural learning process is being interfered with at an early stage. If you have a child who cries a lot, the first and most important priority is *not* to blame yourself. It is no reflection on your ability to cope or how good you are as a carer. Lots of children who have CP cry more than the average child.

My own child was very, very quiet until he was taken off barbiturates at 4 months old. It then took a further four months to get through the desperate screaming which followed and only began to be alleviated when we found an exercise programme which gave him the opportunity to explore fully the world around him. Every family's experience is different but there is one need which all of our children have in common – a need to understand the world around them. The only way to be sure that they get the maximum opportunity for this is to offer them stimulation as often as possible which is appropriate to their age. In addition to this, a child who has restricted mobility needs help to gain access to the world through movement. If they cannot move by themselves we need to move them. If a small baby who has CP doesn't seem to notice you, this is all the more reason to make yourself noticeable. Wear bright colours and make sure there is plenty of light. If he does not seem to respond to sound, play him lots of music and make sure he hears lots of everyday sounds. If he does not move voluntarily, take his arms and legs and give them a chance to feel the world. If he seems very sensitive to touch, kiss and touch him a lot. This will have to be done gently but it is important that he overcomes any sensitivity of touch so persevere. Eventually he will be able to tolerate touch and come to appreciate it.

There may be some alternative remedies which can aid sleep or stimulate action. These are discussed further in Chapter 5.

## Colds and chest infections

It is common for children with CP to have a rather fast and shallow breathing rate and many are susceptible to colds and chest infections. Also, some children may find it difficult to cough up mucus either because they have an inefficient cough reflex or because the shallow breathing allows the mucus to lie on the chest.

There are various ways to deal with these problems. A physiotherapist may be able to suggest some exercises which will encourage deep breathing. Preventative action you can take using alternative methods is dealt with in Chapter 5. Conventional medicine tends towards treatment rather than prevention but there are a number of inhalers and drugs (antibiotics) which may be prescribed by your GP or consultant if your child gets a chest infection. You should not delay in getting treatment for your child if she has a chest infection. Antibiotics have a swift action and can stop an otherwise serious complication in its tracks. Even alternative practitioners will usually advise that you use conventional medicine such as antibiotics rather than risk your child becoming seriously ill with consequent interruption to her overall treatment.

Basic preventative action in the home includes ensuring your child is wrapped up warm if you are going out, keeping the atmosphere at home as dust free as possible, avoiding draughts in the home and maintaining a good diet high in vitamins and low on dairy produce (which tends to be mucus-forming).

## Constipation

Constipation can be one of the most incapacitating minor problems encountered by the young child or adult with CP. It is essential that you find a way to keep the bowels moving. If possible, methods should be found which will not further weaken or damage the intestinal tract. Strong laxatives are the worst for this and the child can become reliant on them. There are a number of readily available preparations which are made from natural substances that do not do permanent damage to the intestines. 'Fybogel' is a good example and can be bought over the counter or obtained with a prescription from your GP or consultant. Preventative measures include close attention to diet, gentle massage (in a clockwise direction) on her tummy, just below the navel, at regular intervals and especially when she needs to go. There are a number of herbal preparations which can be given to help avoid constipation (see Chapter 5). Changes to diet may help. If all else fails suppositories, which are glycerine based and comparatively unharmful, will encourage bowel movement if your child is 'bunged up'. You should not administer suppositories as a matter of course but they can be used very effectively on an occasional basis without doing any long term damage.

There may be certain foods you should avoid or could give more of to ease constipation. For example, roughage in the diet, plenty of fruit (especially plums or prunes), adding olive oil or ground sesame seeds or linseeds can all help. You may need to take care not to give your child too many dairy products as these can be binding. Ensure that your child gets sufficient liquid and drinks with her diet; a dietitian can advise on the appropriate amounts.

The following recipe for easing constipation was given to me by a speech therapist. I have used it successfully with my own son.

---

**Ingredients**
- A 300 gram tin of prunes (stoned) plus the juice
- 3 large, ripe bananas
- Half a pound of mixed dried fruit (or half a pound of dried apricots if preferred)
- 200 ml water

**Method**
Liquidise the ingredients and divide into 10 portions which can be individually frozen.

The sauce can be put on breakfast instead of (or as well as) milk, used as a drink or (if too thick to be used as a drink) offered as a pudding. You should begin by offering the child 15 ml per day of this recipe and work up to a regular consumption of 100 ml per day. Expect to wait up to a week for results.
The recipe is sweet and very tasty.

---

## Otitis media (glue ear)

Otitis media is a common, minor ailment which can affect disabled and non-disabled children alike. Many children without disability have been wrongly thought to have developmental delay because of this condition. It is an infection of the middle ear which may have a serious effect on the child's hearing due to the production of fluid 'glue' in the middle ear. It is slightly more common in pre-term infants than those born at term. Children who have CP may have long term problems with hearing due to brain damage. On the other hand, otitis media can occur in addition, and quite separate to any brain damage but have a further, unnecessary, disabling effect on the child. If you can't distinguish the sounds that are going on around you *and* you have restricted mobility the situation could be very frustrating. It is already difficult enough to make your way through the developmental maze without the added complication of a curable infection. It is vitally important that you get your child's hearing checked regularly as otitis media is much more difficult to pick up in a child who has CP. There is sophisticated machinery available which can detect this condition fairly easily so that treatment can be rapidly administered. If the condition is severe it may require surgery for the insertion of grommets. Some parents as professionals believe that grommets should only be inserted as a last resort as they may increase the possibility of infection and prohibit certain activities such as swimming.

## Slow growth

A significant number of children who have cerebral palsy do not grow as quickly as non-disabled children of the same age. In many cases doctors are unable to explain this. However, two identifiable causes, 'failure to thrive' and growth hormone deficiency, are both treatable.

**Failure to thrive**   This is a general term used by professionals to describe a child who is not growing properly, the cause of which may be poor nutrition. The classification is not specific to children who have cerebral palsy; many children who have no other disability are considered to be failing to thrive. There are a number of reasons why a child may appear to fail to thrive, particularly if the child has a severe physical disability.

Failure to thrive is sometimes assumed to be rooted in problems in the early relationship between mother and child. Emotional deprivation, physical neglect or abuse and withholding of food are commonly associated with this condition. It is also acknowledged in professional circles that the condition of cerebral palsy may, in itself, produce failure to thrive. Many children who have cerebral palsy have immense problems with the physical action required to eat. If the carer has constraints on her time (and even if she doesn't), it may be very difficult to get the child to take in enough food to sustain him.

The best advice I think parents of children in this situation can be given is to ensure that the child receives a well balanced, nutritious diet, and plenty of exercise to complement it. If feeding is so difficult that you cannot get your child to take in sufficient quantities you may wish to consider alternative ways of ensuring he receives enough nutrition. Your consultant should be able to help with this. A referral to a dietitian as early as possible can help with sorting out the best, calorie-filled food to give your child which he can easily accept. I have found supplementing Danny's diet with concentrated protein drinks helpful (these are available from any chemist). Also, adding banana or avocado and cream to the normal diet piles on the calories. If pressure on the family makes it difficult for the main carer to give the necessary time and attention to feeding, then social services should be contacted with a view to providing some help to carers. In practice this is by no means automatic and probably highly dependent on the area you live in.

**Growth hormone deficiency** This is very rare. Sometimes there is brain damage which affects the mechanism which instructs the pituitary gland to release the growth hormone. There are tests which can be carried out for this (although it involves a number of blood tests and possible admission to hospital for a short period). If there is found to be a deficiency of growth hormone in the body there is an option to give growth hormone treatment.

## Behavioural disorders

It has been suggested (by Rutter and colleagues in 1970) that children with brain damage (evidenced by cerebral palsy or epilepsy) are 4–5 times more likely to have behaviour disturbance than non-disabled children. It is thought that such disturbance is not necessarily connected to the brain damage. The enormous pressures and stress put on the family and the child who has cerebral palsy may affect behaviour. There is often a lack of adequate counselling, information and practical assistance when it is immediately required in the early stages of discovering that a child has cerebral palsy. Comments from carers in my own survey suggest, overwhelmingly, that families feel unsupported and ill-informed by the helping professions. The child may, understandably, feel frustrated by lack of mobility and muscular movements which refuse to obey the child's intention. It is difficult for parents to know exactly how to introduce the normal disciplines appropriate in child rearing when they may be having difficulties understanding their child's early communication and be distressed to witness the child's frustration. All of these things may contribute towards the development of behaviour disorders.

The current medical thinking is that such disorders should be, as nearly as possible, treated in the same way as they would be in treating non-disabled children who have such problems.

I would venture to suggest that some of the treatments and therapies which are offered to the child with cerebral palsy could, in themselves, contribute towards the child developing behaviour problems. Professionals, for example, will often openly discuss a child's condition and prognosis, in negative terms, while the child is sitting in the room.

Some therapies require that the child spends long periods of time carrying out activities which are quite unnatural, such as lying face down over someone's lap for long periods of time. There has to be a balance struck between the need for appropriate exercise and the need for the child to experience ordinary life as it can be lived.

Specific treatment for behaviour disorder will depend on its exact nature. There are basically three approaches available. One involves drug therapy, another is behaviour modification using reward systems for appropriate behaviour and a third, less commonly available option, is some form of psychotherapeutic counselling either for the carer, the child or the whole family. With this latter option the family can together examine the problems that they are having and, with the help of a trained therapist, identify causes and explore solutions.

## Hyperactivity

This means that the child is excessively physically active. In children with cerebral palsy this is often known as hyperkinesia. Hyperkinesia describes this condition when the overactivity of the child is related to that child's development. The main characteristics are restlessness, impulsive behaviour, poor concentration span, difficulty in attending to what is being said or going on around them. On occasion, such children may be aggressive, anxious, poor eaters, have difficult sleeping patterns and social and learning difficulties. Children with this condition are not necessarily more active than the average child but their movements are likely to be less purposeful. Given the difficulty of interpreting the meaning of intentional movement in many children who have CP the diagnosis of hyperkinesia is not an easy one to make.

There are a number of ways in which hyperactivity can be treated. A structured environment which includes plenty of time for relaxation may help. Over-stimulation should be avoided (this is very difficult to achieve if your child has other difficulties calling for extra stimulation to help overcome them). Positive reinforcement (i.e. rewarding the child for behaviour which is calm and controlled) may help. There are drugs which can be used to control the effects of hyperactivity but they all have side-effects and these must be weighed up before administration, especially considering that a child with CP already has a number of other disabling experiences to grapple with and may require medication for these which might conflict with the medication prescribed for hyperactivity. The most commonly prescribed drugs are dextro-amphetamine and methylphenidate. These drugs modify the disturbances in attention span, concentration and impulsive behaviour. Side-effects of the drugs, in the short term, can include anorexia, abdominal pain, insomnia, drowsiness, headaches, nail biting, sensitivity and tearfulness. Long term effects may include increased heart rate and growth suppression. Balancing the medication for hyperactivity is quite difficult and needs to be monitored carefully by your consultant.

It is very difficult to isolate hyperactivity as a specific problem relating to cerebral palsy. A restless and frustrated response to the world is quite understandable if you have a condition which makes it difficult for you to communicate or move in the way you want to. Consideration should be given to whether a child is exhibiting a natural reaction to a frustrating situation before hyperactivity is assumed.

## Microcephaly

This is a defect in the growth of the brain as a whole, and is due to damage to the brain which restricts its ability to grow. The brain may be as much as 25 per cent underweight and it is possible that the frontal lobe will be the most severely affected although this is variable. The forehead tends to slope markedly backwards and the ears may appear disproportionately large. Microcephaly tends to be associated with intellectual impairment. Microcephaly must, however, be distinguished from small head size which is also common in children with cerebral palsy. There is no known treatment for microcephaly.

## Hydrocephaly

This is a build up (beyond the normal) of the cerebrospinal fluid within the skull. The main symptom is usually a gradual increase in the size of the upper part of the head out of proportion to the face or the rest of the body. Hydrocephalus has historically been associated with birth fatality or low intellectual progress. However, treatment has become much more successful over recent years. The most common treatment is to implant a valve (known as a shunt) which drains off excess fluid. The problem with the implanting of shunts is that they can cause infection, or may become blocked, and further exacerbate the condition.

## Epilepsy

Epilepsy is a fit of sudden consciousness loss often accompanied by convulsions and/or sudden jerky movements. There are different types of epilepsy which are of varying severity and effect. Up to half of the children who have cerebral palsy are likely to have one type of fit or another either on an occasional basis or at regular intervals. Epilepsy is a common condition irrespective of other brain damage and thought to affect up to 290,000 people in England and Wales alone.

The main categories of epilepsy are: grand mal, petit mal, infantile myclonic seizure, myclonic and akinetic seizures and Jacksonian epilepsy.

**Grand mal**   This is a generalised convulsion which starts very suddenly with twitching of muscles and localised spasms. A general seizure (involving the whole body) often follows. Sometimes there is a warning of an impending fit such as irritability, headache or stomach pains. The face is often distorted, the head thrown back and air expelled from the lungs. There is a danger that the patient might bite their tongue. This usually lasts for 20–40 seconds. The patient then usually collapses into unconsciousness. On waking he may well have severe headache and confusion.

**Petit mal**   These seizures consist mainly of a temporary loss of consciousness. They may be accompanied by a rolling of the eyes, nodding of the head or slight quivering of the muscles. These seizures may appear as 'dizzy spells' or temporary absences, often no longer than 30 seconds in duration. The patient is not likely to collapse but may drop anything he has in his hands and temporarily lose contact with whatever activity he is engaged in.

**Infantile myclonic seizure**   This commonly occurs in infants before the age of 2 and is usually expressed as a sudden dropping of the head and flexion of the arms. Attacks are likely to take place many times in one day. It has been suggested that up to 90 per cent of children with this type of epilepsy are likely to have learning difficulties.

**Myclonic and akinetic seizure (myclonic jerks)**    This type of epilepsy may occur in isolation or in association with other epilepsies. A single group of muscles is usually involved and there may be a sudden loss of postural tone. If the child experiences myclonic jerks frequently it has been suggested that they might interfere with learning.

**Jacksonian epilepsy**    This type of epilepsy frequently involves isolated groups of muscles and consciousness is often retained throughout. Some patients who have Jacksonian epilepsy develop into grand mal patients.

*Diagnosis and treatment of epilepsy*
Diagnosis of the type of fit your child is experiencing is usually obtained through electroencephalography (EEG). This is carried out by a machine recording the spontaneous electrical activity in the brain by placing electrodes on specific points on the scalp and electronically recording events in the cortical and sub-cortical areas of the brain. Different types of epilepsy tend to produce recognisable wave patterns.

## The use of drug therapy

There are a number of instances where drug therapy may be offered to children (and adults) who have cerebral palsy. Most common are those offered to control convulsions and those for relief of tension and muscle spasm. In addition drugs may be offered to relieve constipation, help with sleep, reduce anxiety, reduce hyperactivity and to ease pain after operations.

Great care must be taken when the decision to offer drugs is made. It is necessary to ensure that the dose is right, that it can be maintained within safe limits and also that there are no other preparations on prescription which might adversely interact with what is being proposed.

**Drugs used to control convulsions (anti-convulsants)**    Any general depressant of the nervous system will decrease or abolish epileptic fits but the ones used to treat epilepsy have been selected because they reduce excessive stimulation in the brain without depressing vital centres (such as the respiratory centre) and without sending the patient to sleep. The cause and type of epilepsy must be established before treatment is offered. The selection of the most appropriate drug and dosage is critical and it may take several months to get a patient's symptoms controlled on a particular drug. It is essential that patients follow instructions for taking these drugs exactly and adverse side-effects should be noted and reported to the prescribing doctor.

The dose of an anti-convulsant drug often needs to be slowly increased over time as the body builds up tolerance. This means that the drug becomes ineffective as the body gets used to it. Unfortunately the level of drug in the system which is toxic does not change. This means that the higher the dose is increased the nearer the patient gets to having toxic levels of the drug in his system. When this happens the patient may have to be switched to another anti-convulsant. The change over must be carried out very slowly, as should withdrawal or decreasing the levels of drugs. This is because sudden withdrawal of anti-convulsants can have marked and dangerous effects – which may include anxiety, restlessness, trembling, weakness, abdominal cramps, vomiting, hallucinations, delirium, fits and even death.

Driving and operating machinery needs to be avoided if the patient develops drowsiness as a result of taking these drugs. Some anti-convulsant drugs reduce the effectiveness of oral contraception and there is a slight risk of abnormalities being produced in babies if taken during pregnancy.

Frequent blood level monitoring should be carried out at the beginning of treatment until the patient is stabilised.

Children require more regular and higher dosing than adults as they break down the drugs more quickly. Multiple drug therapy (combining more than one anti-convulsant) should be avoided as this further complicates monitoring and increases the risk of adverse side-effects from the interaction of drugs. The effects of alcohol combined with the effects of anti-convulsant drugs can sometimes be dangerous.

**Drugs used as muscle relaxants** Care must be taken when administering muscle relaxants to take account of any other regular drug use (such as anti-convulsants) as there is a high possibility of muscle relaxant drugs contradicting other drugs.

Diazepam (Valium) is a popular muscle relaxant. Baclofen (Lioresal) is also becoming popular. Dantrolene sodium (Dantrium) used to be popular but its use is gradually diminishing.

**Table 3** Drugs and their side-effects

| | Name of drug | Possible side-effects |
| --- | --- | --- |
| Common anti-convulsant drugs | BARBITUARATES:<br>– Phenobarbitone<br>– Methylphenobarbitone | Confusion when in pain, drowsiness, some dependence, affects enzymes in liver |
| | BARBITURATE RELATED DRUGS:<br>– Primidone | Drowsiness, ataxia, nausea, vertigo, headache, thirst, visual disturbance, anaemia |
| | HYDANTIONS:<br>– Ethotoin<br>– Phenytoin | Can irritate lining of stomach, so must be taken with plenty of fluid. Dizziness, nausea, skin rashes, double vision, mental confusion |
| | SUCCIMIDES:<br>– Ethosuximide | Headache, nausea, drowsiness, apathy, mood change, loss of appetite, ataxia, skin rashes, parkinsonism, difficulty looking at bright lights |
| | BENZODIAZEPINES:<br>– Clonazepam (Rivotril)<br>– Clobazam (Frisium)<br>– Diazepam (Valium)<br>– Lorazepam (Atican) | Drowsiness, fatigue, drooling, difficulty co-ordinating movement, convulsions<br>Drowsiness, fatigue, ataxia, dry mouth, excitement and aggression, constipation, incontinence, trembling |
| | OTHER DRUGS:<br>– Beclamide (Nydrane) | Stomach upsets, dizziness, nervousness, skin rash |
| | – Carbamazepine (Tegretol) | Dryness of mouth, nausea, diarrhoea, dizziness, double vision |

**Table 3** continued

| | Name of drug | Possible side–effects |
|---|---|---|
| **Common anti-convulsant drugs** | – Sulthiame | Loss of appetite, loss of energy, ataxia, breathlessness (in children), sensation on face, hands and feet, nausea, dizziness, loss of weight, mental changes, abdominal pain, drooling, insomnia, blood disorder, increased fits |
| | – Sodium valproate (epilim) | Nausea, stomach upsets, transient loss of hair, oedema, blood disorders, liver damage, occasional death |
| **Common muscle relaxants** | DIAZEPAM (Valium) | See above |
| | BACLOFEN (Lioresal) | Nausea, drowsiness, fatigue, depression, skin rashes; should not be used if patient has a history of epilepsy |
| | DANTROLENE (Dantrium) | Transient drowsiness, dizziness, weakness, malaise, fatigue, diarrhoea; should not be given to children if spasticity serves a purpose, e.g. in walking |
| **Postoperative analgesia for children** | PETHIDINE | Lift in mood, dizziness, sweating, dry mouth, nausea, vomiting, constipation, retention of urine |
| | MORPHINE | Nausea, loss of appetite, constipation, vomiting, confusion, mood change, drowsiness, restlessness |
| | DIAZEPAM (Valium) | See above |
| | NARCAN | Nausea and vomiting |

*Sources:* Peter Parish (1987), Eugene E. Bleck (1987)

**Drugs used to decrease anxiety**   Diazepam (Valium) and related drugs are those principally used to treat anxiety. It belongs to the chlordiazepoxide drug family which has four properties: sedative, anti-anxiety, muscle relaxant and anti-convulsant (see Table 3 under anti-convulsant drugs for common side-effects).

**Drugs used to aid sleep**   Drugs in this group depress brain function; in smaller doses they are used as sedatives (to calm patients down) and in larger doses as hypnotics (to send patients to sleep). They are all habit forming so that patients may quickly become dependent on them. This can be made worse by an increase in restlessness at night when the drug is withdrawn. Tolerance can develop and the side-effects may include anxiety, irritability and depression. They should not be mixed with alcohol. They may impair learning, affect concentration and produce confusion.

**Drugs used to control hyperactivity**   Stimulants are used to control hyperactivity. These drugs and their side-effects are discussed in the previous section on hyperactivity.

**Drugs used to ease constipation**   These are called laxatives and care must be taken not to use them too regularly. They should never be taken to relieve abdominal pains, cramps, colic, nausea or any other symptoms even if associated with constipation.

A high fibre diet, with plenty of fluids, is the most natural way to treat simple constipation. This is achieved by increasing the indigestible waste products in the diet by eating more fruit, leafy vegetables and by adding bran to the diet.

There are very many preparations on the market but there are four main categories of laxative: stimulant laxatives (bisacodyl, cascara, castor oil, danthron, fig, senna, sodium picosulphate); saline laxatives (magnesium sulphate, magnesium hydroxide, sodium sulphate, sodium potassium tartrate, potassium bitrate, lactulose); lubricant laxatives (mineral oils, dioctyl sodium sulphosuccinate, poloxamer); and bulk forming laxatives (agar, tragacanth, ispaghula husks, sterculia, bran).

Stimulant laxatives increase large bowel movement by irritating the lining and/or stimulating the bowel muscles to contract. They may cause cramps, increased mucus secretion and excessive fluid loss. Side-effects vary enormously from person to person.

Saline laxatives increase the bulk of the bowel by causing it to retain water. They take fluids from the body and can cause dehydration, and should therefore be taken with large drinks of water. Lactulose may cause nausea, diarrhoea and wind.

Lubricant laxatives soften the faeces. Mineral oils such as liquid paraffin should be used with extreme caution as it interferes with the absorption of vitamin A and vitamin D and can be dangerous if accidentally inhaled.

Bulk forming laxatives increase the bulk content of the bowel which stimulates the bowel to become active. They must be taken with plenty of fluids to avoid the risk of bowel obstruction.

When faeces are impacted, laxatives administered rectally may be useful. A number of preparations are available, the most harmless of which are probably glycerol suppositories.

**Drugs administered post-operatively** The main drugs used during a hospital stay involving any kind of operation are analgesias or muscle relaxants to relieve pain. Amongst the most commonly used are Pethidine, morphine, diazepam (Valium) and Narcan. As with many other drugs care must be taken to take account of any long term drugs the patient is on in case there are contraindications of their use together with particular analgesias.

**Alternatives to drug therapy** Alternatives exist for all drug therapy but patients and parents should be careful about turning to alternatives. It would be extremely unwise and potentially dangerous, for example, suddenly to take a child who has epilepsy off anti-convulsant drugs because you had discovered a herbal alternative. If you want to try an alternative you should ensure that it is under the guidance of a well-qualified alternative practitioner and that you discuss slow reduction of anti-convulsants with your doctor first. An alternative practitioner may well advise that you maintain your child on anti-convulsant drugs but that he might be able to help you to keep the dosage at a low level by complementing drug therapy. Also, some alternative treatments have adverse side-effects, although they are unlikely to be as severe as those experienced under conventional drug therapy.

Complementary/alternative treatments are discussed in some detail in Chapter 5.

# 3

# Management of cerebral palsy

## Formal treatment and services

This chapter will be divided into a number of sections to cover the various professional forms of assistance which can be offered either by the National Health Service or privately. The chapter is intended to help carers to understand the rationale behind the behaviour of professionals who are providing assistance under a medical model, to enable you to make informed decisions regarding options for treatment, and to provide information about where to go to get it.

These days the medical profession is moving away from the idea that they treat cerebral palsy and towards an idea that cerebral palsy is to be 'managed' by means of setting goals for a child and then carrying out activities aimed at achieving what professionals term 'function' in given areas. The reason for this is that medical professionals have become convinced, after some 50 years of intense efforts to treat cerebral palsy, that the condition cannot be cured but that 'function' can be improved with careful 'management' of a child. The order of priority may often be as follows: communication, activities of daily living (life skills), mobility and walking. It is also now being recognised that hand function is in fact as important (if not more so) than walking. However, different therapists may have different views about what constitutes the main priority to contribute towards optimum, long term function. In practice therapists from different disciplines will be likely to come in and advise on their specific area of expertise with the paediatric consultant taking the lead on priorities.

Health care for children who have disabilities is theoretically commonly organised by a multi-disciplinary team (MDT) based on friendly co-operation between various professionals. Team meetings are held at regular intervals where the progress of individual children will be assessed. This is the most commonly adopted system in Britain. Various criticisms have been made of this system of organisation. There tends to be a fragmented approach where each professional dwells on his or her particular expertise rather than a joint effort to support the child's global development. The team leader (often a consultant) may tend to lead discussions and have an overriding control over methods of treatment and, as team meetings are based on reporting work which has been done with the child, there is a tendency to be backward looking rather than having a positive, goal directed approach.

The interdisciplinary team (IDT) is forward looking, works closely together and is goal directed. Members of the team meet to agree goals a child should be able to reach and ways in which they can co-operate towards attaining those goals with the child. Some authorities in this country are attempting to carry out treatment under this method.

The transdisciplinary team (TDT) is also goal directed and is based on the integration of expertise so that any one member of the team is able to do the job of another member of the team. Under this system one professional can become the main link with the family and build up a close relationship with family and child. This system is virtually unheard of in Britain. The Peto inspired conductive education method practised in Hungary operates on this principle.

The following example demonstrates how these three approaches may differ in relation to self-help in feeding. Under the MDT, feeding might be seen as the domain of the occupational therapist (for appropriate equipment) and the speech and language therapist (for developing appropriate eating patterns). These professionals might give the child self-help practice in specific therapy sessions but, morning and evening, she may be fed (possibly with and possibly without encouragement of self-help) by parents (or house parents in institutions). The IDT might see bringing the spoon to the mouth as a goal. A programme will be discussed to help the child reach this goal and different members of the team will contribute towards this goal during therapy. The occupational therapist might suggest feeding aids which will make the task easier, the speech and language therapist may be able to suggest types of food and communication at meal times which will enhance success, the physiotherapist might suggest ways of encouraging good motor patterns to enable the child to control movement in the task. Under the TDT, training is similar for all members of the team; each is taught to consider all aspects of a child's function and environmental needs. Once the goal is established it easily becomes incorporated into the therapeutic routine of the day.

It may be worth finding out from your consultant or health visitor what kind of teamwork approach is carried out in your area.

## Assessments

During your child's life there will be an ongoing round of assessments made by one or more professionals each with a specific purpose in mind. Some assessments are carried out by members of the team responsible for your child's health care and treatment and some may be carried out at specialist centres.

The consultant may lead the local team in routine assessments on a regular basis with the aim of monitoring progress and making adjustments to a child's treatment pattern. In any case individual therapists who see your child regularly are likely to be carrying out regular assessments of their progress even if only informally.

You may be referred to a specialist centre. You might, for example, get a referral to a communication aids centre to assess your child's needs in regard to the most suitable equipment to help her to maximise the effectiveness of her communication or a seating clinic where your child can try out various aids to improve her posture when seated. At one of these centres there is likely to be a brief assessment undertaken by a multidisciplinary team of professionals working within the centre. They may then produce a report on their observations of your child's abilities and give recommendations regarding the particular need they have been asked to address.

There is a compulsory assessment procedure which takes place if the decision is made by the local education authority that your child needs a statement of special educational needs before entering school or while he is at school. This is usually led by an educational psychologist but reports will be requested from all professionals who have regular contact with your child (see Chapter 7 for more details about this procedure).

Throughout their school life, children who have statements will have their statements regularly reviewed and this will involve regular re-assessments.

When a child with a statement is nearing school-leaving age an assessment will be made of their abilities and needs with regard to further education and possibilities regarding employment.

Individual professionals will make assessments of your child's abilities and needs in regard to their particular area of expertise as and when they feel it is appropriate to do so or if they are asked to do so by another professional.

If you have a need for specially adapted housing or some adaptations in the home an assessment will be made by an occupational therapist to establish adaptations needed and they will report to the local housing authority.

Adults seeking employment can be offered assessments from various organisations dealing in work opportunities for people with disabilities (see Chapter 8).

Assessments of any sort invariably lead to reports being written and distributed to other relevant professionals. In some cases copies of reports will also be sent to the family but this is by no means certain. It is possible, in fact highly likely, that a vast amount of information about your child will be collected and distributed which you will never see, let alone get an opportunity to contribute to, and which will have a direct effect on the kind of options offered to him.

You are often entirely reliant on the goodwill of individual professionals as to whether you are invited to see or contribute to reports written about your child. Thankfully, the law does provide some protection in regard to educational assessments as partnership with parents and the right to see reports is now written into the law.

The effects that reports, passed on from professional to professional, can have may be extremely helpful in ensuring continuity of care and treatment. However, they may sometimes be detrimental. The attitude of professionals dealing with your child is paramount. The key to good report writing is that your child's strengths should be stressed and built upon first and foremost. The family's account of a child's abilities should be given serious consideration since children will often perform tasks more successfully at home, on their own with the family, than when they are under observation from professionals in a contrived situation in which the professional will be placed under a time constraint. Where difficulties are identified they need to be reported in a way which is not offensive and concentrates on positive action which can be taken to overcome obstacles, wherever possible using the child's strengths to enable this. All aspects of the child's life should be taken into account when a report is compiled rather than a concentration on isolated factors. For example a report from a physiotherapist on good positioning which fails to take account of the seating which is available to the child may fall short.

## Action you can take to influence assessments

- In the week leading up to the assessment make a note of everything your child achieves which you think may have some relevance to the assessment and report this to the professionals.
- If you feel able, write your own assessment of your child's abilities and needs and present copies to the professionals who see your child.
- Ask to be sent a copy of any report which is written. The Access to Health Records Act 1990 entitles patients to access all medical records made from 1st November 1991 onwards. However, some GPs have discretion if parents request access to their children's medical records in that they need to be satisfied that access is in the child's interests.
- If you receive a copy of a report and there are aspects of it which you do not feel happy with, write to the professionals concerned voicing your concerns.
- Involve support from within the Disability Rights Movement. There are a number of organisations which concentrate on the need to protect disabled people from unfair treatment and, in some instances (particularly in education) advocates can be made available who will represent you and your child in an official capacity (see the list of useful addresses and contacts on pages 219–231).
- Ask for a second opinion. However, consultants called in to offer second opinions often know and respect the first consultant and may be unwilling to contradict him. Also, assumptions about a child's abilities are often made on the basis of statistics associated with types of CP rather than an open minded assessment of that particular child. This could lead to a consensus of opinion amongst consultants which does not necessarily relate to your own, individual child's development.
- If you can get access to a video camera, regular recording of your child when she is demonstrating her abilities, and any

problems she might have, can help professionals to get a more complete picture of your child. Some support groups now have video cameras which they hire out very cheaply or free. If you need to rent commercially it can cost between £20 and £40 for a day. Purchasing a video camera costs anything from £400 (second hand) to £2000.

There is a great deal of controversy about the best treatment methods for children who have cerebral palsy and individual therapists are bound to have their own opinions and preferences from the wide range of options. Quite often these opinions will be rigid and you may feel pressured to ignore systems which do not find favour with your therapist. You may even be made to feel that to take a different line would be irresponsible.

## Professional roles within the National Health Service

The rest of this chapter outlines the roles of the various, individual professionals you are likely to come across and examines some specific therapies.

### *The health visitor*

The health visitor is a state registered nurse (with extra training as a health visitor and possibly in midwifery) who specialises in mother and child health in the community, especially in the very early days of a child's life. Her responsibilities include:

- Establishing a relationship with the pregnant woman during the antenatal period;
- Visiting the mother and baby in the home to note the family circumstances and give advice on aspects of baby care such as feeding and immunisation;
- Identifying families who have special needs;
- Running sessions at the child health clinic or GP's surgery;
- Health education;
- Visiting play groups and nurseries;
- Liaison with hospital units and links with voluntary bodies;
- Membership of and contribution to the local, multidisciplinary team dealing with children who have disabilities.

The health visitor is often the most vital link between the family in the home and all other services. She is likely to be the first point of contact you will make in the home. It will often be the health visitor with whom you will discuss your concerns in the first instance. Her training should enable her to help identify where a child's development is not following normal patterns.

Being involved with the family from very early on, the health visitor is best placed to provide early advice and act as a liaison point between the hospital, the GP, other Health Service professionals and the Education Service. She can often help out by making referrals for assessment etc. if you are worried and in need of other professional advice.

## The special needs health visitor

In some health authorities one or more health visitors will take on a special role in supporting families in which there are children with disabilities. This facility is not very widespread but, where they exist, special needs health visitors play a vital role in acting as a contact point between the family, the hospital and the community services. They should be equipped with knowledge, not only about your child's disability, but also about the various statutory and charitable sources of support which are available. Ideally, they will also be able to form a link between hospitals where your child's problem may be initially identified and the community health care which you will come to rely upon to some extent. They also should be able to offer counselling (or advice on where you can go to get counselling) and put you in touch with other families so that you can get support from people in a similar situation early on.

## The district nurse

Most community medical practices have a district nurse attached. Otherwise your local hospital or GP can advise you on who to contact. The district nurse can offer help with incontinence (such as the provision of nappies or other continence aids). They can also help to provide supportive mattresses for children who might be in danger of getting pressure sores from lying in one position for any length of time. Basically, the district nurse can be called upon to offer support in any of the nursing care functions which are relevant to your child. If they can't help directly they should be able to refer you to the appropriate professional.

# The paediatric consultant and registrar

The paediatric consultant is a senior doctor who has chosen to specialise in the medical care of children. A paediatric registrar has also chosen to specialise in the medical care of children and is a qualified doctor but at a more junior level than a consultant. The paediatric consultant or registrar will probably be the first specialist you meet when you are aware that your child is not developing to your expectations. Consultants and registrars are based either in hospitals or in community health care practices.

The role of the consultant and registrar is to assess your child's physical condition, to provide a diagnosis where possible, to offer appropriate medical treatment to alleviate any difficulties your child is having and to refer your child to other specialists where there is a problem outside the scope of her own specialism.

The early stages will probably be taken up with the consultant or registrar trying to establish how your child is developing physically against what is considered to be normal development (see the table on pages 25–27 for normal development profile).

# The special care unit

The majority of children who have CP will not have experienced obvious problems at birth and their condition is only picked up as they are developing. If a child has serious problems at birth (such as lack of oxygen) the consultant may be concerned, initially, with guarding against such dangers as further brain damage from fits, failing heart, lungs, kidneys and other organs. If it is thought necessary the child may be monitored in a special care unit where specially trained staff can monitor his heart rate, breathing and other bodily functions. If a baby is born very pre-term he will need to be cared for in the baby unit for many weeks.

If a child is experiencing severe convulsions (fits) at birth precautionary measures may be taken immediately to reduce the risk of further brain damage. Stopping violent fits is a priority and certain drugs (such as phenobarbitone and/or phenytoin) can be administered. These are likely to control fits and may occasionally produce severe side-effects such as extreme drowsiness. The effects of such drugs can make it very difficult for consultants to establish the extent of damage at this point. Another common precaution is to put children in special care on ventilator machines to help with their breathing. This involves assisting the child's breathing by placing a tube through the mouth or nose into the trachea (windpipe). The child might be assisted with early feeding by milk being given through a nasogastric tube which passes through her nose and directly into her stomach.

Thirty years ago, before these early interventions were possible, many babies died who would survive today and many more suffered brain damage who manage to avoid it today. Care needs to be taken when administering intervention. It has been shown that ventilators can cause chest infections, tube feeding can inhibit normal feeding patterns and barbiturates can cause children to become lethargic, depressed and unaware of their environment. As a parent you do not have the medical training to discern whether the treatment being administered is actually necessary or not. You have to rely on the judgement of the consultant. What you can do, however, is to ask questions. Get the staff on the unit to explain why they are taking certain measures, whether there might be negative side-effects and why they feel the importance of the intervention outweighs the side-effect. Try not to be aggressive in your questioning. The staff are genuinely concerned with the welfare of your baby and a relationship of trust between staff and parents is essential.

There will come a point where attempts are made to reduce the child's dependence on these supports and to try and introduce normal patterns. This can be a slow process requiring much patience and persistence especially if you are trying to introduce sucking at the breast or bottle. The staff at the hospital should be trained to help mothers to establish normal feeding. Even once feeding is established the baby might take a lot longer to drink the required amount of milk than a child who is not disabled would do. Great care needs to be taken that the child receives enough nutrition right from the start. Help may be available from a breast feeding counsellor through the National Childbirth Trust and from your health visitor as well as the staff in the unit.

## Children attending outpatients

In the majority of cases the condition will not have been picked up at birth and the child may not begin to make regular visits to the consultant until she is some months old and it has been established that she is having some problems.

Children who have been supported in the special care environment are likely to be discharged home with their parents or into another caring environment. Carers/parents may be asked to continue to administer drugs or portable ventilation at home and the child will probably visit outpatients on a regular basis so that the consultant can monitor her progress.

For children who are attending outpatients, one of the consultant's concerns will be to establish whether infant reflexes are staying present beyond the age when they should have disappeared, whether they appear to see and hear and how their muscle tone is developing in addition to organ function (heart, lungs, kidneys etc.) It is very unlikely that the consultant will tell you that they are looking out for signs of cerebral palsy. In cases where there has been an obvious incident this might be because they want to be sure of their facts before they confirm or allay your suspicions. If the referral has come from a parent they will be waiting for the evidence of their own eyes and possibly even offering reassurances that there are no obvious signs of a problem while they deliberate about your child's developmental pattern.

The doctor will be interested to note whether any deformities seem to be developing and how the muscle is developing. Possible signs to watch out for include the following:

- Subdislocation or dislocation of the hips, varus and spine;
- Inequality in length of legs;
- Fixing of joints detected when they are put quickly through a range of motion;
- Head and trunk flexion (curled up in a foetal position), extension (head and trunk thrown backwards) or rotation (head or trunk twisted to one side or the other);
- Shoulders flexed (bunched up), extended (thrown back), abducted (turned outwards) or rotated (turned in);
- Very tight muscles (increased muscle tone or hypertonia);
- Very loose muscles (reduced muscle tone or hypotonia);
- Unco-ordinated or jerky movements;
- Lack of visual or auditory attention;
- Frequent spasms (presenting as sudden, jerky movements).

## Getting the diagnosis

During my own research I found that 63 per cent of respondents had to ask before they were given a diagnosis and that those 63 per cent felt that information was withheld from them. In addition, 61 per cent were dissatisfied with the answers to their questions after diagnosis was given. In almost all cases the questions were answered by a consultant.

It is very important not to fall into the trap of blaming the consultants for this apparent breakdown of communication between them and carers. Cerebral palsy is very difficult to diagnose and it is even more difficult to predict the outcome of any specific case.

'She may have brain damage or developmental delay', is often the first indication a consultant will give. As mentioned in the introduction, however, it is impossible for the consultant to predict accurately your child's future from early symptoms. There are even cases where babies seem to be extremely affected physically but appear to make complete recoveries. As time goes on, and if symptoms persist, a consultant may venture to suggest a diagnosis. In addition to cerebral palsy your child might have other complications.

As your child gets older the consultant will be looking to see if any contractures (restriction of joint movement) or deformities (such as curvature of the spine) are developing. It is possible that your child will have been referred to physiotherapy and occupational therapy for appropriate advice on ways of handling and on equipment which can reduce the likelihood of these conditions occurring. This is discussed further on in this chapter. The consultant may also refer your child to a speech and language therapist who can advise with feeding, speech, communication and language development. Referral to a speech and language therapist tends to be slower than to other therapists. If you feel your child would benefit from a speech and language therapist's input you are entitled to self-refer.

There are particular, key areas of the body where consultants will be concerned to ensure that abnormality does not persist. Muscles in the arms and legs go in pairs. It is often the case (especially in spastic CP) that one of the pairs will become stretched while the other becomes weakened by this. Neck muscles and back and chest muscles can stretch or become very loose which may lead to the bones which the muscles support going out of shape. There is particular concern to avoid deformity of the spine and hips (which can easily become dislocated) which would create a great impediment to walking. The tendon at the back of the foot (known as the Achilles tendon) can also present severe problems by shortening and pulling the feet out of proportion.

## Surgery

Medical research suggests that a child will have reached full walking potential by the age of 7. This is not necessarily always the case. There are many reports of children acquiring the skill of walking after this age. Surgery to improve gait (patterns of walking, standing and balancing) is not generally recommended until a child's lower limb potential has been fully assessed (perhaps by the age of 4, 5 or more). Upper limb surgery is not usually advised before the age of 6 or more so that selective control and sensation can be assessed first.

Many surgeons would prefer to see contractures avoided and gait and upper limb mobility improved through good physiotherapy. However, there are still numerous instances where surgery is advised. Most surgical procedures involve shortening, lengthening or cutting muscles which are causing bones to distort and severely affecting a patient's ability to function. Instrumentation is also used. This involves the insertion of a rod next to deformed bone to straighten it. The cause of deformity lies not so much in spastic muscles but in their opponents, which are often weak. The key to successful surgery rests on a sensitive appraisal of the effect any procedure might have in other areas of the body. Many incorrect postures are used to compensate for a fundamental or causative deformity elsewhere. Surgery on the secondary deformity runs the risk of further disabling the patient by removing compensation she may need in order to function. Total gait and posture analysis is advised therefore before any surgical procedure is contemplated.

Many surgeons feel that a child must be motivated to benefit from surgery and must have an intelligence level which will enable them to understand the procedures they will be undergoing.

### Major problems and complications which might arise through surgery

- Not all spastic states are produced by cerebral palsy. For example, some metabolic diseases cause spasticity and surgery may not be appropriate in these cases. Accurate diagnosis is essential therefore.

- Apparently weak muscles may have hidden strengths which could be removed by surgery.
- Timing is essential. In the first 3–4 years of life it may not be possible to establish where the main problems will occur. Ambulation (walking) might be difficult to achieve through surgery after the age of 8. Multiple surgery (correcting a number of deformities in one operative procedure) avoids repeated hospitalisation and anaesthetic but it might be less effective because of the difficulty in evaluating eventual muscle balance.
- Goals must be correct. Surgery to the extremities (feet and hands) may not be effective if hip and spine deformity are central to the lack of balance.
- The willing co-operation of patient and parent is fundamental. Whether or not procedures are painful or causing frustration must be taken into account. Patient and parent should be involved in planning for corrective surgery and made totally aware of the purpose and likely outcome of the procedure.
- Any surgery is likely to involve lengthy pre- and post-operative care. The application of splints and/or plastercasts are commonly needed. There will also be disruption to education caused by time spent hospitalised and convalescing.

Corrective surgery may be suggested in the following cases. This is not an exhaustive list but represents the more common surgical procedures:

**Spinal deformities**
*Scoliosis*   Where the spine has distorted sideways in an S curve – instrumentation (implanting rods) and spinal fusion are sometimes used in this case;
*Thoracic kyphosis*   Where the upper spine has distorted so that the patient has a very rounded back;
*Lumbar lordosis*   Where the lower spine is distorted producing convexity in front – this can cause extreme lower back pain but might also be a compensatory deformity developed as an adaptation to hip flexion;

**Pelvic deformities**
*Increased posterior inclination*   Where the pelvis protrudes at the rear;

*Increased anterior inclination*   Where the pelvis protrudes at the front;

*Pelvic rotation*   Where the pelvis is twisted horizontally;

*Pelvic obliquity*   Where the pelvis is distorted at an angle making one thigh appear higher than the other.

**Hip deformities**   This is the second most common orthopaedic problem in CP (scoliosis being the first). Hip dislocation is the most serious deformity of the hip which can occur. The severity of the hip deformity can be assessed by examining the extent of hip abduction (measured by the distance achievable between legs when held apart); 20 degrees abduction is considered very severe, 35–40 degrees moderate and beyond 40 degrees mild. Normal hip abduction is approximately 80 degrees. It may be possible to avoid dislocation by regular passive abduction through stretching or splinting but this is often supplemented by surgical treatment at some time.

**Knee deformities**   Knees are often not straight enough or too straight. This might be secondary to a hip deformity so care should be taken if surgery is being suggested that the primary deformity is being taken into account. Surgical procedures often involve weakening the hamstring muscle.

**Foot and ankle deformities**

*Equinus*   This is caused by shortening of the Achilles tendon producing a distorted appearance to the foot. Surgical procedures are available to 'lengthen' the contracted muscle.

**Hand and wrist deformities**   The infant 'thumb in palm' reflex commonly persists in CP and 'fisting' is common. Also, the wrist may become flexed (bunched up) or extended (stretched back). There are a number of procedures which may help to correct hand and wrist deformities by shortening or lengthening certain muscles.

**Plastercasting and splinting**   These procedures may be used post-operatively or, in some cases, instead of surgery. Plastercasting can be used to reduce tone to help avoid contracture but it fails to improve function because the immobility of the limbs in plastercast can further weaken muscles. Splinting is a procedure of holding limbs in place with splints. This procedure may be used post-operatively. Children often find splints uncomfortable and may be expected to sleep in them.

If surgery is suggested it is essential that the consultant is questioned closely on the purpose and alternatives. If you are not fully satisfied ask for a second opinion.

Guy's Hospital is developing a gait analysis system which involves substantial input from physiotherapists and an analysis of a child's total muscle involvement and use.

Surgical procedures often involve an increase in drug use.

## Specific therapies
### *The team of therapists*

In most areas the team of therapists (known as paramedics) will consist of a physiotherapist, an occupational therapist and a speech and language therapist. How early any of these therapists get involved in your child's treatment needs will depend on the number of therapists available in the area, the severity and nature of your child's disability and the cohesion of the referral system in your area. My research suggests that the physiotherapist is likely to see all children who are diagnosed or suspected of having cerebral palsy. Other therapists are likely to be brought in as and when and if their input is considered necessary.

The therapists will all be interested in your child's development but from different perspectives. The physiotherapist is most concerned with the development of your child's movements (motor ability), ensuring that deformity and contractures do not occur and that preventative measures are taken regarding dislocation of joints. The occupational therapist will be primarily concerned with the development of your child's ability to help herself and with advising which appliances and equipment can support this. The speech and language therapist concentrates on your child's language and communication development. All three are likely to use development check lists based on 'average, normal development'. There is no such thing as a standard normal rate of development. Every child is an individual and no child follows an exact developmental pattern but there are certain milestones (activities such as 'sitting up unaided', 'rolling over from back to tummy') which tend to occur at roughly the same age for most children.

## The physiotherapist

A referral to the physiotherapist is often the earliest referral made. The job of 'the physio' is to help a child's mobility to develop normally and to carry out and teach exercises designed to avoid contractures and bone deformity and unwanted movement.

Physiotherapists are sometimes able to offer exercises which will help to reduce spasm in children that experience it, quite common in medium to severe situations. They may also be able to suggest exercises to improve breathing patterns.

There are very many different techniques which can be applied by physiotherapists. In general, they are trained to work with your child to enable her to obtain maximum physical function but this can be done in a variety of ways. Physiotherapists receive very little paediatric training. Traditionally, physiotherapy has concentrated on isolated areas of dysfunction and worked on the area where dysfunction occurs in an attempt to eliminate it. This is because physiotherapy often tends to be applied to people who have a temporary, rather than a permanent disability. For example, if someone has a broken arm, there are certain exercises which can be carried out to help the person regain function in the broken arm more quickly than he might have done without exercise. However, cerebral palsy is more complex than this. It is a permanent disorder which is caused by a dysfunction of the brain rather than the limbs and muscles. A physiotherapist working with a child who has cerebral palsy has to recognise that this child will probably need to carry out some form of exercise for most of her life. These days physiotherapists tend to specialise so that they are likely to be aware that they are dealing with a long term problem which will require constant monitoring.

Certain equipment is the remit of the physiotherapist. There is often a grey area between the role of the physio and the occupational therapist in regard to certain equipment but a physiotherapist could be expected to get involved in the provision of standing frames, wedges, adapted bikes and trikes and other mobility/posture aids which have a direct effect on a child's physical progress and support.

## Conductive education and physiotherapy

Ester Cotton is a physiotherapist who has been very involved in the conductive education movement and has had considerable influence in bringing this type of training into Britain. This is discussed in detail in Chapter 7 under education; I will not dwell on this technique in this chapter because the approach is very different from mainstream physiotherapy and not considered, by those who practise it, to be a therapy so much as an educational process. Conductive education approaches cerebral palsy as a learning difficulty. The central philosophy of conductive education is that a child who has cerebral palsy has a learning problem which may be overcome with repeated practice of everyday activities carried out in an environment which is, as nearly as possible, like the environment the majority of children grow up in. Wheelchairs and other adaptations are avoided if possible and the child learns all of the activities necessary for living from one person who is trained in all of his needs; mobility, communication and pre-school play. This person is called a 'conductor'.

## Bobath physiotherapy

This is a very popular 'early intervention' method (also known as neurodevelopmental treatment – NDT) because it attempts to inhibit unnatural reflexes and movements from the time they arise. Treatment is thought to be most effective if started as soon as there is any indication of a suspected diagnosis of CP. Professor Bobath (a medical practitioner) and his wife (a physiotherapist) were developing this method for some 30 years up until their recent deaths.

The Bobath technique seeks to eliminate the infant reflexes which persist in a child who has CP but which normally disappear after a short period of time. Examples of this are: the tendency small babies have to 'fist' their hands, a tendency to turn the head in the opposite direction when they reach out with the opposite arm, head constantly thrown back.

The treatment programme consists of passive positioning of the child in postures devised to reduce spasticity. At the same time it tries to give the child a sensation of normal movement (for example, by facilitating the automatic righting reaction) and implementing the stages of normal development from rolling, through sitting, kneeling, crawling and standing to walking. In recent years, however, the Bobaths concluded that they had been overrating the importance of the abnormal reflexes in assessments and that the normal development sequence does not have to be followed too closely.

It is central to Bobath that skills in handling the child to enable the best possible posture and mobility are transferred to parents so that they can be aware of this throughout the normal day.

Nancie Finnie (a physiotherapist and a strong supporter of this method) has written a book called *Handling the Young Cerebral Palsied Child at Home* which explains ways of handing a child in the day to day home environment that will help to inhibit 'abnormal' motor patterns.

The Bobath Centre in London offers free assessment and treatment to British children through referral from a paediatric doctor. There is a 3–6 month waiting list. Another Bobath centre has been opened in Wales (see useful addresses, p. 219).

## *The occupational therapist*

Occupational therapists are trained to look at self-help and appropriate equipment which will be likely to enhance or promote self-help in the child. They become involved in helping their clients to have appropriate adaptations made to the environment in which they live to facilitate independence, as well as assisting clients in adapting to their environment.

Some children who have CP will not need specialist equipment. For those who do, the occupational therapist may get involved in any of the following activities: advising on the best cups, spoons etc. to enable easy feeding, providing seating (or adapting existing seating) to give your child maximum support, lending or suggesting toys to aid develoment, providing or suggesting suitable pushchairs (or adapting existing ones), advice on wheelchairs, walking frames, standing frames and side lying boards and adapting equipment a child uses in everyday life to suit his physical developmental needs. Additionally, the occupational therapist is trained to suggest appropriate adaptations to the home and community to facilitate independence.

Unfortunately, resources tend to be very limited and this is reflected in what most occupational therapists can offer. You need to be satisfied that your child's buggy offers sufficient support to avoid any damage being done to their posture.

Some children are fine in an ordinary buggy. For others a buggy can be made more supportive with creative use of foam. Some children will benefit from a specially adapted buggy. Unfortunately, many of the commonly available special buggies don't fold and are very bulky. Some double up as car seats but this is not very helpful for those who have to rely on public transport. The convaid cruiser is a rather bulky buggy but at least it will fold. The Kelly from Ortho Kinetics is another folding buggy which suits children who need some minimal support. The MacLaren Major buggy is very lightweight and easy to fold. On its own it does not offer very much support but a supportive insert can be obtained from Smirthwaite Ltd (see useful addresses p. 219). The Snug seat can be used as a fairly supportive buggy and a car seat. Some children not walking may be expected to continue to use buggies well beyond an age it would normally be appropriate. Wheelchairs can be offered to young children but they are difficult to get and tend to come in standard issue which may not be appropriate to your child's individual needs.

There are a great variety of special chairs but it is very difficult for therapists, let alone parents, to get a comprehensive overview of what is available.

When you are considering your child's seating needs it is important that you get a clear idea of what you're hoping the special seating will achieve. Some seating is very bulky. Many special seats have trays in front of them which mean that the child is unable to join the rest of the family at the dining table. Many chairs available on the market depend on numerous straps to hold the child in place. I don't think I would have been very comfortable as a child if several parts of my body were strapped down every time I sat in a chair. On the other hand, chairs which do not rely on straps probably require the child to put in some effort to keep their posture correct. Thus sitting down becomes an activity requiring work rather than one of relaxation. If your child clearly needs special seating it might be worth considering the option of more than one chair, perhaps one for relaxing and one for active sitting. It is unlikely that your local authority will fund more than one chair however.

There are a number of centres which specialise in seating and your occupational therapist may be able to get you a referral to one of these centres if she is not able to come up with a

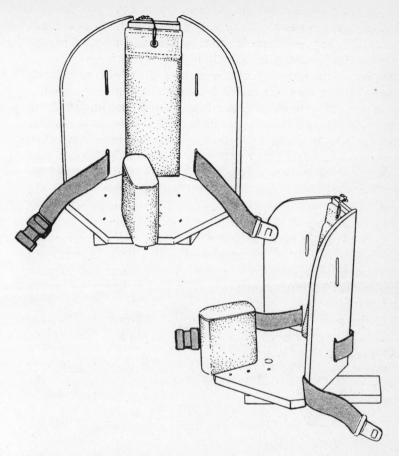

*The Rifton Corner Seat is very useful for sitting and playing at floor level. A strong cardboard box can also be adapted.*

satisfactory, standard solution (see the list of useful addresses and contacts on pages 219–231).

It is often considered important for children to stand for a period of time each day. This is because taking weight through the feet helps the proper development of the hip joint which, in turn, helps to prevent dislocation. If a child is unable to stand without support there are a variety of standing frames available. Other ways to help a child with standing practice include holding them in a standing position, giving them some support with your hands while they lean on a sofa or low table and helping them to hold on to a bar or ladder backed chair while they are in the standing position. Not all children will be able to manage these more independent ways of standing but for those who can there is the added benefit of achievement through their own efforts.

Toilet seats and supportive potties can help a child to develop important independent function.

As a child gets older and bigger, adaptations in the home might be needed. These could include hoists and grab rails for bathing, special beds which you can lower and raise to facilitate dressing, ramps and stair lifts.

My research suggests that only about 54 per cent of parents whose children have cerebral palsy receive advice from an occupational therapist, and only 32 per cent of these see one after their child has reached the age of 2.

If you really want to review the options for yourself a fairly wide range is on view at the Naidex Exhibition which is held twice a year, once in London and once in the middle or north of England. The magazine *Disability Now* published monthly from the Scope office advertises these events well and does a helpful review of each one. At these exhibitions you have the opportunity to see an item, possibly try it out and talk to representatives from supplying firms about your particular needs. You can then ask your own therapist to arrange for an assessment of items you are interested in. Some firms are willing to come out with equipment even if you are not able to involve a therapist, but you need to be sure that you feel confident about your child's physical support needs if you are 'going it alone'. Alternatively you can see some examples of equipment at a specialist centre such as the Disabled Living Foundation (see the list of useful addresses and contacts on pages 219–231).

## Speech and language therapy

The speech and language therapist is primarily concerned with a child's communication. Communication is a two way process so a speech therapist will be just as interested in how much a child can understand as how much they can communicate to the outside world. They are concerned with establishing how a child understands language, whether he can understand verbal instructions or whether he needs clues from his environment to understand what is going on around him. The speech and language therapist will be concerned to give the child some means of communicating to the outside world within his particular capabilities. This might be through activities which encourage speech, signing, electronic aids or picture boards may be used. Sometimes the use of extra aids to speech (like signing) will support the development of vocal communication.

Children with cerebral palsy (even in mild cases) often tend to be slow in developing verbal communication. Research has shown that children who are helped to communicate using appropriate aids are often more successful at developing speech as well.

Speech and language therapists often get involved in helping the child with feeding as it is believed that good feeding patterns are helpful for the possibility of developing normal speech. This is because the same muscles are involved in both activities.

**Alternatives to verbal communication** The main system for signing (using symbolic language through hand movement or indicating symbols on a board) which is available for young children in this country is known as Makaton. This is derived from British sign language which is one of the most commonly used signing languages for adults in this country. The Makaton system is also available in the form of sign boards which can be used for children to point to the symbol to indicate their choice. The system can also be loaded onto a computer. In addition there are picture cards which go with the system to enable an adult to teach a child the meanings of the different signs and symbols.

Other commonly used symbol systems include: the Bliss symbolic system, the Rhebus system, and the Mayor Johnson, picture communication symbols. I personally favour the latter of these because they are clear, representative drawings with a written word underneath to aid reading development and are adaptable for use at a variety of ages and ability levels. However, some teachers and therapists would argue that other symbol systems offer a greater opportunity to develop a flow of language and sentence construction as communication becomes more complex.

There are also a large number of systems which allow the child to convey ordinary speech through some kind of techno-logical aid. The Possum is one of the longest running aids of this kind.

**BABY**

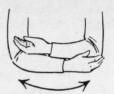

Mike cradling a
baby in the arms
and rocking

**BICYCLE**

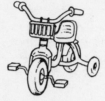
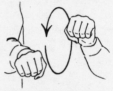

Two fists held a
few inches apart
make peddling action

**BIRD**

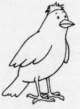
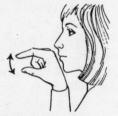

Index finger and
thumb open and
close in front of
mouth like a beak

**BISCUIT**

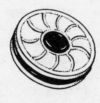
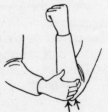

Fingertips of right
clawed hand tap near
left elbow twice

*Examples of Makaton signing*

**DRINK**

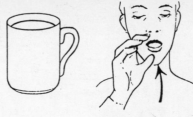

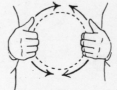

Mike having a
drink

**TREE**

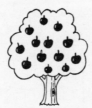

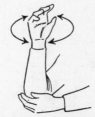

Right elbow cradled
in left hand. Right
clawed hand palm
up/left twists from
side to side

**CAR**

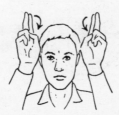

Mike holding and
moving a steering
wheel

**RABBIT**

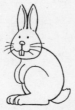

Palm forward 'N' hands, held
at either side of head, bend
several times to indicate ears

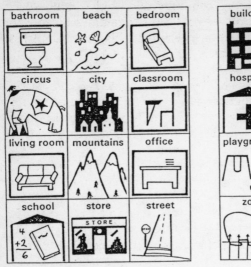

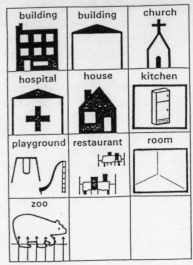

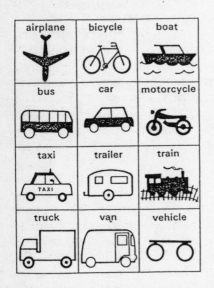

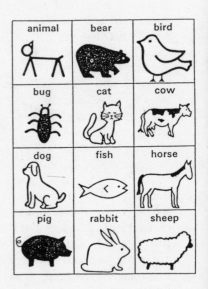

*Examples of Mayer – Johnson Symbols (© 1981 Mayer – Johnson Co.)*

There are a number of communication aid centres where children can be taken to test out, and sometimes borrow for trial purposes, various communication aids (see the list of useful addresses and contacts on pages 219–231).

If children are at all delayed in speech acquisition and/or hand function it is a good idea to investigate switch-operated toys and communication strategies from as early an age as possible. Even if a child is going to acquire speech later on such devices give them early access to two-way communication and some control over their environment.

On the most fundamental level, every child should be encouraged to develop a way of saying YES and NO. This might be through mustering whatever movements they can to indicate these two. My own son uses a raised eyebrow for YES and a very light leftward movement of the head for NO. Another child I know of opens her mouth to say YES and keeps it closed for NO. Some children can manage a nod of the head and a shake, others can use a two switch system, either operated by head movement, hands or even feet. These two simple words can give a child access to the world of communication and choice, and a tremendous boost to their self-confidence, as long as those with them are prepared to offer a range of options and be creative enough to keep on going until they have elicited the child's desired response.

Initially, it might be worth offering one switch only which will turn a toy on or off (with perhaps the added facility of a latching box which will serve as a timer and facilitate the switch having two functions). This will acclimatise the young child to the notion of 'cause and effect'. Very quickly however, the majority of children should be moved on to two switch use where they can control two different activities or make a choice of two outputs. The Four-talk is a box which allows you to record any 1–4 statements (depending on how many switches are being used) over and over again for the child to access. The Echo-4 has a similar function. Even this can become quite limiting for the non-verbal child who is eager to communicate. Then it is worth thinking about one of the more sophisticated machines which have a voice output, such as Dinavox, Liberator, Macaw, Chameleon (also a computer), Alpha Talker, or other similar devices.

Some of these machines can vary the amount of output between one phrase or word (using the whole screen as a switch) and anything up to 30 or more using sections on a screen. Children who have difficulty pressing a particular, small section on a screen (perhaps because of difficulty with fine hand control movements) may be able to learn to scan and select from a large set of options using only one switch. There is a switch for everyone, whatever their difficulty with control over movement. Some operate on the lightest movement; some can be activated only by a muscle twitch or the interruption of a beam of light or even by only blinking.

If you are having difficulty getting information about such aids through your speech and language therapist you can see a range of this kind of equipment at the Naidex Exhibition which is held twice a year and most manufacturers will willingly come into your home to give demonstrations. Some firms will lend equipment for a small fee or free of charge so that you can really try it out to see if it works for your child.

It is difficult to get an early assessment of your child's needs in this respect because electronic communication aids are very expensive and still not a statutory right for children with communication difficulties. Don't give up. If you feel your child would benefit from such a device press for an assessment and, if necessary, a re-assessment of their needs and then press your health or education authority to provide for your child's needs. The facility is there if you can persuade providers that the benefit will be worth it (see useful addresses on p. 219 for places to go for advice).

For children who have real difficulty with movement as well as speech there are a number of ways in which they can be helped to communicate more effectively. One of these is with sensible and sensitive use of facilitation. In other words, you offer physical support to your child to inhibit spasm or unwanted movement or to relax tight muscles to give them a bit more control or freedom of movement in order to allow them to move their arms to fist or finger point. As time goes on and they hopefully become more able to make the required movement independently, support can be gradually reduced until they are independent communicators. I have certainly used this method very successfully with one child who is now able to communicate in a quite sophisticated way without any physical support.

The method known as Facilitated Communication has a lot in common with the method I have just been describing. This method has received a great deal of support and opposition because it assumes that the child cannot communicate without some physical help. Critics maintain it is the facilitator who is communicating and not the child. This may be true in some cases but there are very many valid examples of children learning to make clear communication for the first time using this method. If your child is having difficulty making himself heard it might be worth contacting one of the centres who offer this kind of training (see useful addresses p. 219). A good trainer in Facilitated Communication has the child's eventual independent communication as a prime goal and it can offer a real confidence boost to a child who is crying out to communicate.

**Computers** The advent of computers has opened up new and exciting possibilities in communication for people who are physically restricted and unable to communicate vocally. In addition to being a fast and efficient communication aid the computer can be a tool for facilitating early learning.

Contrary to popular belief, computers can be appropriately used to stimulate even very young children (less than one year old). There is a very wide variety of software (which means program of games etc.) available to help teach young children. Many of these teaching programs will have a useful purpose in complementing the speech therapist's work on language development.

For very young children and/or older children who have very little mobility there are numerous switches which can be obtained which will enable the operator to use the computer with the lightest of touches and minimal movement or fine control.

At the most simple level programs are available which enable a child to get an idea of 'cause and effect', for example the child presses the switch or touch pad and something exciting happens on the screen. Possibilities range through simple tasks such as picture matching-up to proper sentence construction etc.

Computer and communication aids are different. A computer is a guide to learning while a communication aid is an opportunity to get your message across. However, the two do overlap.

**Communication for children with visual impairment** If a child has restricted mobility and visual impairment the carers and the speech and language therapists are set a challenging task to enable communication. It is very important to bring other senses (hearing, touch, taste and smell) into play with communication. The first level of communication is to enable a child to make choices and this could be done through many media. Examples include the following:

- Certain fabrics or other touch sensitive items which the child can relate to a desired object or activity. By touching the appropriate item the child can indicate choice.
- Making the visual clue very distinct and clear. This can be achieved either by using very contrasting colours or by using different fluorescent or reflective colours and/or shapes.
- Combining the hearing with touch. When the child hears a certain auditory clue they can press the appropriate indicator for their choice.

**Communication for children with hearing impairment**   As with visual impairment the other senses (i.e. vision, touch, taste and smell) will assume greater importance to provide compensation.

If the child has enough fine motor control of her hands she should be enabled to start learning sign language at as early an age as possible. Even if she is unable to sign you can help to make your communications clear by signing to her and being generally physically expressive.

Sound can actually be felt through vibration even by someone who is completely deaf. Make sure she gets every opportunity to 'feel' as well as see things, especially items which have a sound element to them.

Ensure she gets the opportunity to maximise learning through vision. Lots of books and other visual learning aids will help.

If the hearing deficit is sensory neural (i.e. part of the brain damage) it may be possible to stimulate improvement in hearing by presenting the stimuli of sound.

**Communication for children with dual sensory impairment**
This is generally taken to mean impairment in both hearing and vision. In this case the sense of touch plays a vital role in communication. The organisation SENSE has been set up to support people who have dual sensory impairment and can offer advice on special teaching techniques to facilitate communication.

## Peripatetic teaching

There are some areas where peripatetic teaching is available for your child from a very early age. A good peripatetic teacher can help you and your child to find ways of providing necessary stimulation within the constraints of her physical disability. Some teaching systems have an integrated approach in that they view physical disability as a learning problem to be overcome alongside other developmental milestones (see Chapter 7). Even if your child is still very small there are educational opportunities he may be able to take advantage of (such as the portage system) so you are advised to read Chapter 7 even if your child is still very small.

A good peripatetic teacher can be a great complement to the work being carried out by the speech and language therapist.

## Under fives provision

It is well worth finding out if there are any mother and toddler groups in your area. If you want your child to have an equal place in the community, integration needs to begin very early. Giving your child the opportunity to meet and play with non-disabled toddlers who live in the locality is a good starting place. It's also an opportunity for you to get out and meet other mums with small children. So often carers of small children with disabilities become isolated and this isolation can be passed on to the child.

It is also worth finding out whether there are any under fives groups locally who specialise in catering for children with disabilities. Such play groups often have specially adapted toys and playgroup sessions which aim to help your child with her early development. If you do manage to find a specialist playgroup it is still worth trying to get into a mainstream toddler group as well. It will help your child's later integration if she is mixing with disabled and non-disabled children alike from the start.

## The psychologist

Psychologists are employed in the assessment of children who are considered to have special needs with a principle interest in their learning ability, their behaviour and their understanding of the world around them.

Psychology is a science which attempts to base itself on the objective techniques developed in the physical sciences such as physics, chemistry and biology.

It is likely that your child will be assessed at various times by a psychologist, and the psychologist's reports can have a significant effect on the opportunities offered to your child. An educational psychologist may be called in to do assessments on children when entering school, monitor their development within school and provide guidance regarding their further education as emerging young adults. A clinical psychologist or an educational psychologist might become involved with children who appear to have behavioural difficulties.

There is much controversy and debate within psychology on the most appropriate methods to assess ability and behaviour. A widely used method is based on IQ, personality and sociability, which is carried out on the basis of scoring children against a very rigid set of tests. To succeed in these tests children need to be physically mobile, have all of their senses (such as sight and hearing) in perfect working order and to have developed an ability to communicate effectively. The child who has cerebral palsy is immediately put at a disadvantage because she is likely to have limitations in one or more of the areas of function upon which psychology testing is based.

More enlightened psychologists will carry out much of their assessment in a more informal way by observing the child in a natural setting on a number of occasions and over a period of time. They will also talk to the parents to gain insight into the parents' view of their child's abilities.

An educational psychologist is likely to take the lead in assessing your child's educational needs as he approaches school age. It is worth finding out how much the individual psychologist knows about cerebral palsy. If you feel they are not experienced enough you should feel able to challenge their involvement and ask for someone with some expertise in the field. Even if they do have experience, you should feel confident that your involvement and your knowledge about your child will be taken on board.

## Music and art therapy

Both of these artistic media are enjoyable to children and both can be used to support a child's development in a number of ways. Through music a child can express her emotions, develop a sense of rhythm (which will in turn support their physical development), develop their communication skills, benefit from auditory and tactile (through vibration) stimulation and relax. Through art a child can express emotion, improve fine motor control, practise valuable pre-school skills and benefit from the tactile and visual stimulation of different artistic media. These are just some of the benefits.

You don't have to wait until you have made contact with a specialist to give your child experience in art and music. To play music all you need are instruments (home made ones will do) and a casette player. Shakers made of plastic washing up bottles filled with rice, upside-down saucepans and wooden spoons and milk bottle tops on string can provide you with a percussion section. Alternatively you can buy percussion instruments such as maraccas, tambourines and drums. Give your child a range of music to enjoy from classical to pop, nursery rhymes to reggae. To enjoy art all you need is paper, paints, non-toxic glue and a variety of materials (cloth, milk bottle tops, pasta, rice, lentils). Playdough, plasticine and clay can all be used for model building.

You can seek specialist advice in these areas. To find out more about music therapy you can contact The British Society for Music Therapy or the Nordoff-Robbins Music Therapy Centre. To find out more about art therapy you can contact the British Association of Art Therapy (see the list of useful addresses and contacts on page 219).

## Vibro-acoustic therapy

Vibro-acoustics is a treatment system for stiff muscles and impaired circulation. It is a further development of music therapy which combines vibrations produced by low frequency sinus tones with therapeutic music. The patient relaxes in a chair, or on a bed, which has speakers built into it. Half of the speakers emit low frequency sound waves and the other half play relaxing music.

Research trials are underway in the use of vibro-acoustics at Harperbury Hospital under the direction of music therapist Tony Wigram and physiotherapist Lynn Weaks. Initial findings are very promising. Regular use of the treatment appears to reduce high muscle tone, ease constipation, improve vocalisation prospects, reduce spasm and aid general relaxation. The equipment is marketed through Kirton Health Care Group who can arrange for demonstrations of the equipment (see the list of useful addresses and contacts on page 219). However, the equipment is very expensive.

## The role of the social worker

Not all families will have regular, or even any, contact with a social worker. Social workers are employed by local social service departments and it is their job to help families and individuals by providing them with access to practical support in the community. The social worker is also employed to be aware of and keep an eye on anyone who is considered to be vulnerable in their locality and to intervene if their client seems to be in imminent danger.

If a child has disabilities his family may be offered support from a social worker but usually only if there is some other reason to suppose that the family is vulnerable beyond the simple fact of disability. Examples might be single parent families, families where the social services have reason to believe that the child might be being abused or in danger of abuse, families who have had previous contact with social services, or perhaps by self-referral or referral from another professional.

Another role social workers have is to place children in foster care and to organise adoption.

All children who are fostered, adopted or brought up in residential homes will be under the care of a social worker who will be trying to ensure that the child's needs are being met adequately by the arrangements which are being made for them.

The social worker should be able to find out what benefits you are entitled to and how you can go about claiming them although your health visitor may also be able to advise you in this area if you do not have a social worker.

There are social workers attached to each of the six regional offices of Scope who can provide valuable advice and support if you do not have access to a social worker within social services.

## Respite care

A potentially vulnerable situation can be avoided by offer of regular respite care. There are generally two types of respite care available. Either a trained foster mother can look after your child for occasional or more regular periods of time or the same facility can be offered by some residential homes. The main aim is to give the family a break so that they can care more effectively for their child at home. However the majority of families are not offered this facility until their child is older. It is likely that a great deal of stress will have built up by the time respite care becomes an option. Many families would not find it easy to part with their child even for a short while and even when they plainly need a break. This is understandable as the closest members of the child's family will often understand their needs much better than strangers. For this reason it is important to try and arrange respite care where your child will get to know someone and they will likewise get to know her so that you can rest assured she is being looked after to your satisfaction. It is a good idea to make sure the temporary carer has all of your child's particular needs and ways of communicating explained to her and it will help to arrange to go on short visits with your child, at first only leaving her for a short while each time until she has built up a relationship with the carer who will provide respite. If you are not happy with the arrangements being offered it is important that you say so right away so that an alternative can be sought.

It can take many months to establish respite care so it's wise to investigate this option before you get exhausted to breaking point. This service is usually offered through a social worker.

If you are receiving Attendance Allowance (see Chapter 11) your right to it could be affected even if you only receive a small amount of respite care on a regular basis.

## Getting referred to a counsellor

The consultant who sees your child, or your GP, can refer you for counselling or you can self-refer. Basically, counselling involves regular visits to a trained counsellor whose role is to help you to understand, cope with and hopefully overcome any negative feelings you may have about your family's circumstances. It is also an opportunity for carers to have their needs acknowledged. It's often the case that the needs of your child seem so overwhelming that your own can get submerged. The end result of this is often that the stress of submerging your own needs can lead to depression or other health problems.

You might also be able to seek support from a psychotherapist. Psychotherapists are also trained to help you to overcome any negative feelings you may be experiencing but they will be likely to do this in a less directive way than a counsellor. If you self-refer to a counsellor or psychotherapist you may have to go privately and have to pay.

## Systems less widely available through the National Health Service

### *Doman-Delacato: Patterning*

Glenn Doman was a physiotherapist who worked in the late 1940s with Carl Delacato (an educator) and Robert Doman (a physician specialising in physical rehabilitation). A growing body of evidence that sensory enrichment as well as sensory deprivation can alter the structure of the brain, inspired Doman to develop a technique which aims to treat the brain by altering the neurological (the function of the web of tissues and branching cells which support the nerve fibres and cells of the nervous system) system within the brain.

Prior to the introduction of the Doman-Delacato system of treatment there had been an assumption that brain damage was irreversible and treatment centred on inhibiting symptoms of brain damage (such as abnormal movement). The Doman-Delacato principle is that it is possible to treat the brain itself to enable function to be restored naturally through the restoration of the brain's capacity to dictate appropriate function. To put it more simply, this treatment rests on the theory that, when a part of the brain is damaged, other parts of the brain are capable of taking over the function of the damaged area. However, this may not occur naturally and the 'patterning' therapy is designed to stimulate the functioning parts of the brain to develop and to take over the job of those parts of the brain which have been damaged.

There is a fairly well-established theory that development takes place in a hierarchical way. Mobility is perceived to begin with the child on their stomach, reaching out; later on, crawling on their belly; then creeping (up on all fours) and finally pulling themselves up into a standing position. Doman and others (Temple Fay was another leader in the field of the neurological development of the brain) undertook extensive reviews of research into the effect of environmental stimulation on the developing brain. There is a vast amount of research which suggests that the actual structure of the brain is changed and its development enhanced by external factors. For example, crawling has been shown to stimulate the firing of secondary motor neurons in the brain. It has been postulated that babies crawl in order to ensure that the brain develops properly. (Obviously this is not a conscious action but nature sees to it that the activities we spontaneously engage in in infancy will equip us for normal life.) This theory has been backed up by other research which shows that children who have no disabilities but who 'missed out' the crawling stage of development may tend to be slower in certain cognitive areas, such as mathematical ability, when they grow older. Similarly, the tendency children have of enjoying 'spinning round until they are dizzy' and falling over laughing has a very functional purpose. It helps children to develop balance in later life.

The basic principle behind patterning is that mobility is only attained through movement. In addition, where a child has disabilities which interrupt the normal development process, that movement needs to be frequent, intense and repetitive. The Doman-Delacato method also emphasises the importance of sensory and intellectual stimulation as part of a rounded programme of activities tailored to suit the needs of each individual child and maximise their development potential.

The first institute to provide patterning was the 'Institute of Human Potential' in Philadelphia, USA where Doman set up the practice. There are at least three similar institutes now operating in Britain (see list of useful addresses and contacts on pages 219–231).

**How does patterning work in practice?** Initially the child attends the institute (with their family) for a very detailed, two-day assessment. During this time the developmentalists (the name given to the therapists who work in this field) will set out to establish where your child's development seems to have become stuck. The assessment which is produced invariably shows that each child is functioning at different levels in various aspects of development as determined by the nature of the brain damage. For example, a child of 2 may have the hand function of a 3-month old child, the hearing and comprehension of a 2 year old, the sociability of a one year old, the vision of a 9 month old, the movement of a one year old, the speech of a 6 month old and self-help capacity of a 5 month old. A programme of activities is then worked out which is designed to help the child to raise the 'age level' in areas where they are functioning at a lower than desired level.

The programme involves short, sharp bursts of activity to be carried out at very regular intervals, in exactly the same way, for a number of times each day. Activities usually last for 1–5 minutes each and are carried out in rapid succession. Examples of the kinds of exercises include:

- *Masking* (wearing a mask for say one minute which has a valve at the bottom to control oxygen intake and encourage your child to breathe more deeply);
- *Cross pattern* – this involves three people, one on each side of the child and the third person turning his head; the child is then moved through the action of crawling for a specified number of minutes;
- *Walking with ladders* – this involves aiding the child to walk under horizontal ladders, holding onto the ladder above his head to help steady himself as he takes each step;
- *Arm unlocking and hip unlocking* are exercises for stretching and loosening the arms, legs and hip joints;
- *Stand ups* – the child practises standing from a seated position on the adult's lap; the adult is kneeling.

The above are just a very few example exercises. An individual programme is developed for each child depending on their particular needs.

A session will last between half an hour and three quarters of an hour and requires input from up to three helpers to facilitate the exercises.

The programme can only work if the family is able to get help from a number of volunteers who are willing to commit themselves to learning the exercises and coming into the home to carry them out on a regular basis. The institute offers advice on ways to recruit volunteers but a fair amount of resourcefulness, organisation and determination is required of the family. In addition to this you need to become resigned to a rigid routine of a steady stream of people coming through the house for short periods of time to participate. Having support and input from volunteers can be an uplifting experience but, on the other hand, it can become very wearing to be constantly interacting with visitors whatever your mood that day. Patterning can be particularly stressful for 'private' people.

The exercises themselves are rigorous and have to be carried out in the same manner whether or not your child feels inclined to co-operate. It is common for children underoing patterning to protest strongly and this can be distressing for all concerned. A detached approach needs to be developed if your child is not keen on the programme but you feel that the benefits outweigh this.

The institutes generally recommend that you give the programme two years before deciding whether or not it is working. It takes a long time to counter the effects of brain damage no matter what therapy you opt for and you need to give it a reasonable trial period before reaching any conclusions. However, the institute is likely to be the first to recommend ceasing the programme if they feel the child is not benefiting from it. Each child's programme is re-assessed and amended as necessary on a regular basis (2–4 times per year) so there is constant monitoring and evaluation of the effectiveness of the treatment.

The Kerland Clinic (one of the British institutes) has departed slightly from the mainstream of institutes offering this treatment. They believe that children actually require less input in terms of hours on programme to get the same results. Most institutes recommend up to eight hours a day on programme. The Kerland believes that the optimum is 2–3 hours a day. This allows the child time to lead a normal life and to practise the skills acquired through the programme as well as minimising the stress placed on families. They maintain that families on more rigorous programmes often do not carry them out whereas their more realistic programme allows for fuller co-operation between institute and family. They do, however, expect families to adhere strictly to the minimum programme that they produce.

Patterning is one of the most controversial therapies available to children who have brain damage. Support and dissent is vehemently expressed and backed up by a host of scientific data on both sides. There is quite a lot of literature supporting both sides of the argument. Arguments against patterning seem to rest on the stress it can introduce into a family's life and the lack of scientific data to prove the premise upon which it rests. The latter argument I would discount. The study of the brain and the effects of brain damage is so much in its infancy that no-one can truly claim to have established any conclusive evidence to support or disprove any method designed to minimise the detrimental effects.

The stimulation offered through patterning is intense and consistent. Families where a child is very severely affected who have tried patterning often report that they finally feel they are, for the first time, able to really participate in helping their child. The clinics that offer patterning generally have enormous respect for the child whatever the severity of their disability and this can have a very positive effect on family life.

## The Vojta method

Vaslav Vojta developed his approach from the work of Temple Fay. This treatment is most widely used in Germany. The theory behind his approach is that the child with cerebral palsy has the same reflex movements that can be provoked in the non-disabled newborn child. The treatment programme elicits patterns of reflex motion by manual pressure on 'trigger zones' to induce reflex patterns such as creeping and turning. These patterns of motion are then expected to be 'imprinted' in the central nervous system, stored within the brain and thereby allow normal motor patterns to occur. Parents are instructed in the method so that assessment is only necessary every few weeks. Vojta advised that treatment should cease if no improvement is seen within a year of commencing treatment.

## Ayres sensory integrative therapy

The theory behind this method is that children with CP are unable to integrate the sensory inputs (tactile and proprioceptive) from their trunk and limbs. Consequently the vestibular system fails to provide correct information about the movement and posture of the limbs and posture resulting in cerebral palsy. Thus, primitive reflexes persist and the child is unable to plan their motor activity. The treatment is one of passive and tactile and proprioceptive stimulation, which should enable the brain to re-programme and make new connections. The treatment method is mainly based on constant motion stimulation such as swinging in a hammock or on a playground swing or whirling in a swivel chair.

## The Root method

This method attempts to reduce spasticity and activate contraction of weak muscles by tactile stimulation with heat, cold and brushing.

# 4

# Day to day life

This chapter aims to give you useful tips for enabling your child in his day to day life.

## Mobility

Mobility is more than getting from one place to another. It is movement. Many children who have cerebral palsy will have varying degrees of difficulty with movement. For some, walking may be the only problem. For others hand function will be impaired. In more severe cases there may be difficulties in all movement including the movement of the child's head from left to right and up and down, and the rotation of the trunk and pelvis.

There is more than one way to tackle difficulties with mobility. The two main approaches involve working to improve mobility with exercises and purposeful play on the one hand and on the other, making changes to the environment so that limitations in mobility place less restriction on a child's enjoyment of life. The second approach is discussed in Chapter 6.

### Exercises

Your community or hospital physiotherapist may give you an exercise programme which you can carry out in the home. You may also receive training in ways of handling your child to inhibit unwanted movement. If they do not offer this, *ask for it*. The physiotherapist will help the child to achieve much more by teaching his carers how to carry out simple exercises and proper handling on a regular basis. The physiotherapist should also explain the purpose of the exercises so that you know what your aims are and are able to monitor progress. Ask whether your physiotherapist is trained in Bobath. If not, ask her to find out more about Bobath. You can ask your consultant to refer you to the Bobath centre for assessment. Some basic Bobath exercises can be carried out without interfering with your own life too dramatically. For example, while your child is very young you can give her a good stretch at the same time as sitting down watching television. You are likely to have your child on your lap to read stories to her. At the same time you can be holding her in such a way that her posture is being corrected.

In every activity it will be helpful to your child if her posture is taken into account and rectified whether you are walking in the park, playing in the garden, playing in the house or just sitting down in front of the television together. It need not be a chore as, with practice, it becomes second nature to keep your child's positioning and movements stable. As she grows older your early training will hopefully reap rewards and she will become able to self-correct automatically. It is also essential that you teach anyone who is likely to handle your child for any length of time the correct way to hold her. Otherwise you are likely to become frustrated and feel that only you can be trusted with your child. This will only add to your stress.

The first priority for a child who has cerebral palsy is to avoid contractures (permanent tightening or slacking of the muscles) which could ultimately cause deformity (bone structure growing incorrectly). The likelihood of contractures increases with the severity of the mobility restriction. The second priority is to enable your child to move as nearly as possible in normal motor patterns. This will give her the greatest opportunity to feel comfortable and confident.

There are a number of publications which can be obtained through Scope which offer advice to parents on physiotherapy in the home.

## Diet and nutrition

Children with CP are often using a surprising amount of energy even if they are not very mobile. Muscle spasm, for example, uses energy. A well balanced diet is essential for all of us. Many children with CP are likely to have difficulties with eating certain foods because of chewing and/or swallowing problems. If you need practical help your consultant or GP may be able to refer you to a dietitian who can advise on the kind of diet your child needs and a speech and language therapist can advise on the actual method of feeding.

Try to ensure that you separate out the different tastes as your child grows. If she has problems with developing the ability to chew there are techniques you can use to help the development of chewing such as offering dried apricots or fruit straps in between meals. For children who would find these difficult you can still encourage the chewing reflex by allowing them to chew on (but not swallow) a piece of fruit securely wrapped in a piece of muslin which you can control so that they do not need to deal with the swallowing of solid food. If you are able, try to vary the texture of different foods given to your child. For example, I have found that I can give Danny the meat section of his meal with a grainier texture by putting it through a coffee grinder rather than puréeing it. All attempts at varying texture will add to a child's eating development and enjoyment of food.

Make sure that your child has a good balanced diet with proteins (found in meat, cheese or beans) carbohydrates (found in potatoes and bread), roughage (found in oats, wheatgerm and green vegetables), fats (found in butter and oil), vitamins and minerals (found in fruit and vegetables), and plenty of fluids. You should be advised by a health visitor or dietician about the amount of calories your child should receive for his or her weight. If it is difficult to provide enough in the normal way you could consider adding food supplements or fortified drinks to their diet. You can also mix normal foods in a way which increases protein, carbohydrate or fat content without adding too much to bulk. For example, banana, honey, cream and/or egg can be added to a simple breakfast cereal to considerably enhance its calorie content.

## Feeding

Self-feeding can begin as early as 9 months. Small babies automatically bring everything they handle to their mouths. Eventually this is turned into the skill to bring food to their mouths. At first there is no apparent co-ordination to this activity but with teaching from carers, children learn to turn an automatic reaction into a deliberate and quite sophisticated activity. Some children who have cerebral palsy will miss out on these early learning opportunities. They can be helped enormously if their parents are taught to compensate by showing them how to feed themselves from the appropriate age.

To get advice on this one aspect of a child's daily life you may have to go to as many as five different professionals. The physiotherapist will concentrate on the best positioning of your child. The dietitian can advise on the best kinds of food to give her. The speech and language therapist can advise on the best ways to achieve a good chewing pattern and mouth closure. The occupational therapist can advise on appropriate feeding equipment and seating. Finally, you may need to discuss any digestive problems with the consultant. In order to give relevant advice it is essential that these professionals observe your child while she is eating, and it is preferable for them to work together to ensure that they do not give contradictory advice. However, it is not an easy task to gather so many experts together at the right time for such a consultation and, even if you can, it is highly unlikely that a child will be willing to carry on her normal feeding routine with such an audience.

The system of conductive education which is becoming more popular in this country and originated in Hungary involves one professional, the conductor, in advising on all aspects of a child's daily activities. The disadvantage here is that it is not possible for one person covering such a wide range of activities to gain the same depth of understanding in any particular area. At the end of the day it is up to the carer and child to work out the most suitable feeding routine, having taken as much advice from various sources as they can.

Make sure your child can see the plate, the food which is on it and the spoon bringing the food from the plate to her mouth. This is especially important for children with hearing impairment. Talk to her about the process and let her see, feel and smell the food, feel the plate and the spoon and get a sense of their proximity to each other and to her.

Children without disabilities go through a stage when they get very messy during feeding. There is a danger that carers of children who have disabilities will keep their children extra clean either because it is easier to do so because they are not attempting to feed themselves or because the carer feels (maybe even subconsciously) that it accentuates the 'look' of disability.

It is important that you are aware of where the food is ending up. If food is left round a child's mouth throughout a meal it may cause her to lose the sensitivity or the 'feel' for where the food should be. However, there is no harm in a child with disabilities getting the same opportunity to experience food fully by getting her hands in it for example.

It is important to ensure that the child can see the spoon coming to her mouth when you are doing the feeding, and there are various techniques to encourage good chewing and mouth closure which a speech and language therapist or a physiotherapist may be able to advise on. Some children have difficulty keeping their mouths closed and/or have a habit of thrusting out their tongue when trying to eat. Also, children with CP may take a long time to move from the mouth movements associated with sucking from the breast or bottle to the rounded chew required to break down solid food in the mouth. If your child has difficulties with this, the move from the sucking to chewing may need to be encouraged slowly and patiently by very gradually increasing the density of texture and later on the 'lumpiness' of the food offered. Some children with CP have difficulty with their gag reflex. This means that they find it hard to cough up bits of food that go down the wrong way. If this is a particular problem for your child, advice should be sought from a speech and language therapist or your paediatric consultant.

Whilst your child needs your assistance with eating you could give her the opportunity to attempt some self-help with feeding at each meal, provided you are satisfied that she has eaten sufficient food for nourishment. This can be done however severely affected a child is. At the very least you can place a spoon in the child's hand and guide it as far as is comfortable to give her first-hand experience. If she is able to get her hand to her mouth you can guide the spoon all the way. You can also encourage her to pick up food (such as cake, biscuits, bread or fruit) in her hands and bring it to her own mouth. Make sure, however, that such an activity does not contribute to her receiving insufficient nutrition. If in doubt consult a dietitian to ensure that your child is getting an adequate diet before introducing this kind of self-help.

## Breast feeding or bottle feeding the young baby

These days mothers are encouraged to breast feed whenever possible, especially for the first few weeks of a child's life. It has now been established that the very early breast milk contains many different factors which help the baby to build up his natural immune system. Children who have been in special care, tube-fed or even just slow to feed at the breast may have difficulty getting enough breast milk to sustain them. It is possible to feed the early breast milk to the baby via the tube feeding method and milk can be expressed into bottles so that the baby can still benefit from mother's natural milk even if he cannot suck at the breast. It may be possible to supplement breast feeding with commercial preparations. Care should be taken that you do not deplete your supply of breast milk if you are supplementing. The breast needs to be stimulated by regular sucking to enable the production of more milk.

There are breast feeding counsellors in most parts of the country. The National Childbirth Trust should be able to put you in touch with your local breast feeding counsellor.

## Dental care

Children who have CP may be more susceptible to tooth decay than their non-disabled peers. This is because the natural, self-cleaning which is facilitated by saliva (especially at night) may be disrupted. In addition, debris which usually gets moved away by the motion of the tongue may not be cleared so effectively if a child's tongue is less mobile.

Regular brushing of teeth is vital. You should start to clean your baby's teeth as soon as they appear in the mouth. If necessary, there are also fluoride drops which you can get prescribed by your dentist and which can be given to your child last thing at night. When brushing your child's teeth try to develop a technique which is consistent. Work around your child's mouth brushing two or three teeth at a time in a circular or 'mini scrub' motion. Pay particular attention to the inner surfaces and the small, difficult to clean spaces between teeth and the biting surfaces of the teeth at the back of the mouth. Using a battery operated toothbrush might help to make teeth cleaning easier.

Dental treatment can be very distressing for a young child. It is better to prevent the need if at all possible. If your child does need dental treatment there are some dentists who specialise in dental care for children who have disabilities (see the list of useful addresses and contacts on page 219). Alternatively your GP or consultant, or your regular dentist, may be able to advise you of a suitable specialist.

## The importance of hand function

Many children with CP will have no problems with mobility in the upper part of their bodies. However, a significant number do. It is important that your child gets every opportunity to experience the world with his hands. During my own research I found that whether their child would walk was the second most common concern for most carers. Very few respondents noted the importance of hand function. Many professionals and adults with disabilities would contend that hand function is far more necessary for independence than walking. You can get around in a wheelchair if the right facilities (such as ramps and lifts) are available in the environment but it is more difficult to produce mechanical aids which can take over the fine motor role played by the hands.

Encourage your child to use his hands as actively as he can from as young an age as possible. While he is still a baby, make sure he has mobiles and dangling toys to reach out to. If your child has a visual or hearing impairment choose mobiles which also make a sound, are very brightly coloured and, if possible, have different textures.

As the child gets older ensure that he is offered interesting and varied opportunities to use his hands in play. Encourage him to use his hands to play with toys appropriate to his age (with help if necessary) – for example, knocking down and building bricks, playdough. Later still you can encourage him to push, pull and pick up his toys. If your child has very restricted hand movement it might still be possible for him to use his hands to press a touch sensitive switch. A speech or language therapist may be able to assist or you may be able to seek advice from a communications aids centre.

Ester Cotton has produced a very useful booklet called *The hand as a guide to learning* which contains useful programmes to develop hand function (see the further reading list on page 232).

## Play

Play is an essential activity for all children. This is where real learning begins. It may not be easy for some children who have CP to engage in spontaneous play so you will need to be ready to give whatever assistance you can to help them enjoy playing. This is an area where you can fully involve friends and family in supporting you in helping your child to develop.

Because CP is such a varied condition ranging from very mild disability to total immobility it is difficult to prescribe exactly how to be enabling in a general guide like this one. You will need to ensure that your child's toys are readily available, easy to get at and that she has some way of letting you know what she wants to play with at any given time. As she gets older, and depending on the degree of her disability, she will be able to indicate this in a clear and certain way. However, you need to ensure that she doesn't miss out on the early opportunity to make choices in the area of play. As early as possible you need to establish a way for her to indicate preferences. This may be through speech or signs and, later on, through sign boards or electronic communications. If your child is slow to develop speech, a speech and language therapist can help you and your child to find the quickest and easiest method of communication.

The following list of play ideas are graded from the very young upwards. I'm sure there are lots more ideas that you can think up for yourself. A mirror can be a great aid in playing so that your child can get visual feedback on what she is doing. It can even be actively introduced into play by enabling the child to, for example, smear shaving cream on a mirror or blow bubbles towards one.

## 0–2 years

- Play mat and frame with dangling toys;
- Rattles, windmills;
- Rocking and bouncing games;
- Making lots of babbling and cooing noises;
- Tickling games;
- Building bricks – begin with building them up for her to knock down, later on help her to build her own towers to knock down;
- Picture books – you can also get picture books which have the complement of sounds and raised textures to stimulate hearing and touch;
- Hide and seek with toys and people behind curtains/under towels etc.;
- Hitting things – wooden spoons on saucepans for example;
- Imitation and turn taking;
- Playing with mirrors;
- Unwrapping toys (don't put tape on wrapping paper);
- Water and sand;
- Lentils, rice and pasta in tubs to sit in, put your hands in or just throw about;
- You need to be careful to watch that she doesn't put small objects in her mouth that she might choke on.

**1–3 years**
- Posting box games;
- Finger puppets;
- Tunnel games;
- Surprise bags full of toys and interesting objects for your child to find;
- Pulling and pushing;
- Lucky dip;
- Picking correct object from a selection (for example you can ask your child to find you the cow from a selection of farmyard animals);
- Pretend games with dollies and teddies;
- Painting, using fingers or brushes;
- Cars and trains.

**2–4 years**
- Story books;
- Helping round the house;
- Making cakes and other food;
- Ball games;
- Obstacle courses;
- Messy play with a purpose (e.g. sculptures in sand, boats on water);
- Playdough modelling;
- Sticking textures on paper with non-toxic glue;
- Printing (potato prints etc.);
- Spot the difference;
- Shape and colour matching;
- Make believe;
- 'Simon says'-type copying games;
- Toy shops;
- Turning boxes into toys (such as castles, cars or space ships);
- Lego/Duplo;
- Action rhymes;
- Listening games;
- Making music with home-made instruments.

## Seating

Some children who have CP can manage well enough with an ordinary chair. If this is not the case, is your child using a chair which holds her firmly in position but at the same time allows her some freedom of movement in her hands, arms and upper trunk? Good seating is essential for all of us and particularly so for a child who has CP as they may need to be seated more than the average child and many activities will be likely to take place in a sitting position. There are numerous alternatives. Standard special seating is available through occupational therapists but these chairs can sometimes be designed to hold a child firmly in place rather than to allow freedom of movement and therefore only tackle half the needs. You could experiment with ordinary high chairs supplemented with the creative use of cushions and foam padding if needed. For this you will need your local children's store to be willing to let you spend some time experimenting on their premises to ensure that you don't waste your money buying inappropriate furniture. There are seating clinics to which you can be referred which are particularly useful if your child is likely to spend a lot of time sitting down. See the useful addresses and contacts list for addresses of centres which specialise in appliances and equipment, including seating.

## Appliances and equipment

Everyday life poses enormous problems for people who have restricted mobility and movements they cannot control. There is an enormous range of specialised equipment designed to help compensate for this from the earliest age into adulthood. However, the first problem is finding out what choices exist. The second is finding the substantial finance that such equipment often requires. The other major problem is that standardised equipment cannot easily be tailored to suit the needs of every individual. The list given in the table is not exhaustive but is intended to give you an indication of the kind of equipment that exists and whether or not it is likely to be provided free of charge (usually funded by social services). The occupational therapist is the professional who is trained in the use of equipment but she may not have the most up to date information on what is available. Also, equipment which is routinely provided through social services may not be the most appropriate for your particular needs.

There are a number of walking frames available which are not issued through state funding and which might be more appropriate for your child's needs. The David Hart Clinic in Birmingham has designed a walking device which is extremely adaptable and enables even quite severely disabled childen to

**Table 4** Aids, appliances and equipment

| Equipment | Free? |
| --- | --- |
| High chair | Yes |
| Adapted buggy | Not until 30 months (most state-provided buggies are too heavy and will not fold) |
| Baby seat | Yes |
| Foam wedges for exercises | Yes |
| Bath seat | Yes |
| Bath hoists | Yes |
| Potty | Yes |
| Toilet seat | Yes |
| Washing machine | Maybe |
| Walking frame | Yes |
| Wheelchair | Yes |
| Adaptations to toilets | Yes |
| Adaptations to the home | Maybe |
| Stair lifts | Maybe |
| Special beds | Yes |
| Ramps | Yes |

enjoy walking and also to have their hands free for exploration. (See the list of useful addresses and contacts for further information.)

Any wheelchairs available will often be of a standard type. Sophisticated chairs may not be available unless you can fund them yourself or unless you can provide evidence that your child is a special case.

Funding may also be available for special beds (for example, you may need to get a bed which you can lower and raise to facilitate dressing as well as getting in and out of bed).

Examples of adaptations to the home for which you might be able to get funding include moving bedrooms and bathrooms on to ground floor level, lowering the sink and cooker in the kitchen, and lowering light switches.

For all equipment, appliances and adaptations, state funding will depend on assessment and recommendation from the appropriate professional. To be sure you have examined all of the alternatives it is worth contacting organisations such as the Disabled Living Foundation, which specialise in equipment (see the list of useful addresses and contacts on page 219). It has to be stressed that equipment is not made available free of charge very readily. Funding is low for such needs and resources very stretched. If your consultant is willing to confirm that you need a certain piece of equipment it will strengthen your case. Also, there are a number of charities who will consider making one-off grants to provide equipment which you are unable to get through the state system. Your local library will have a list of grant-making trusts.

The Independent Living Fund and the Family Fund (a government grant aid system administered by the Rowntree Trust) may be able to help. Before the Family Fund will agree to provide a grant you will have to be assessed by one of their own social workers but once you are recognised as one of their clients you should find it fairly straightforward to apply for annual grants for special equipment as long as your consultant or therapists agree that you need it and the item concerned is one which would not normally receive state funding. The kind of things you can expect to get funded by the Family Fund include holidays (in this country), driving lessons for carers and washing machines. They normally offer one modest grant per year to families who have been accepted as eligible.

Equipment designed specifically for conductive education is economical, attractive, versatile and comprehensive. While conductive education equipment may not be appropriate for every child it can offer the opportunity for children to maximise their independence and is extremely space saving. A number of firms specialise in equipment but one of the most popular manufacturers is G. & S. Smirthwaite who can send catalogues on request (see the list of useful addresses and contacts on page 219). It is advisable to discuss equipment with an occupational therapist or a physiotherapist before you purchase it to be sure that it will be appropriate for your child.

## *Floor play*

One of the most valuable pieces of advice I ever received regarding Danny's needs was to *'put him on the floor'*. A child's earliest independence comes from exploring the world, using whatever mobility he has, from a position where he is free to do so. Putting a child on the floor, even if he has very little mobility, at least allows for the possibility of exploration. Time spent lying on the floor with a few toys around will be a valuable opportunity to exercise early self-help in play and mobility.

Because our children have special needs we can easily get caught in a trap of thinking that we must always be controlling our children's positioning and activities but *all* children must have the chance to learn from experience. If you are offering a lot of stimulation to your child (input), there has to be an opportunity for him to show you what he has learned (output) by being allowed a free reign occasionally. Putting him on the floor to explore is one way to enable this.

## Stimulating those with sensory impairment

This will not apply to all children who have CP, but many do have disabilities additional to motor disorder. Any of the five senses can be involved in sensory impairment. Severely affected children may begin life with all five senses impaired. It has been found that appropriate stimulation at an early stage can help the child to defeat, or at least to lessen, sensory impairment.

### *Vision*

Cortical visual impairment is sometimes a problem which accompanies CP. It means that the child does not seem to see, or does not seem to see well (due to damage in the visual cortex of the brain), even though the eyes appear to function properly. This is a condition which may persist into adulthood but, in many cases, may recover to some extent. Stimulation of the eyes by using lights and bright colours can be of enormous benefit in helping the recovery process. Ensure that the room is always brightly lit when the child is doing any activity unless you are deliberately wishing to isolate bright objects such as coloured bulbs etc. The following tips may help you to create some enjoyable visual stimulation for your child:

- You could make a play mat out of shiny paper covered with sticky-backed clear plastic (the kind you can buy in rolls for covering textbooks etc.) You can further add to the effect by scattering glitter and other shiny objects under the plastic. You can add squeaky buttons to bring auditory stimulation and pleasure into the game.
- Set up Christmas lights and Christmas decorations on a frame for your child to play under.
- Get an ultra violet light and rig it up in a room where you can cut out other light. Show your child shapes cut out of fluorescent paper under the ultra violet light. There has been some concern that too much exposure to ultra violet can be harmful (such as causing cataracts) so be very careful not to keep her under the light for very long.

- Get hold of some disco lights and let her enjoy frequent light shows.
- Make sure you have a bright light shining on her toys when you are playing with her.
- In Danny's early days he had a lot of success with one of those space blankets used by runners after marathons. They are very shiny, make a noise at the slightest touch and move easily with only a very small amount of manipulation.

## Hearing

If your child has sensory neural impairment which has some potential for recovery, sound may still play a central role in activities.

- Ensure that a visual or tactile clue accompanies all sounds which are presented to stimulate hearing. Toys which vibrate as well as sound are helpful. If you place your hands on a speaker you will feel the reverberation of the sound. If you play a drum, the vibration can be felt as well as heard. Disco lights which flash in time to the music can help your child to develop a sense of rhythm.
- It may help to judge as well as stimulate a child's hearing if you gradually reduce the volume of a piece of music in a play session.
- Be expressive when you communicate. Use sign language as well as speech even if your child is not learning to communicate with signing.

## Sensitivity (or lack of) to touch

Some children with CP will start life very sensitive to touch or seemingly lacking the full sense of touch.

- Hugging and kissing is a nurturing and effective way to begin the process of desensitisation. Some children will not like to be touched at first but, if you persevere, they are likely to overcome this.
- Toys and books which explore different textures are readily available from shops such as early learning centres and may be helpful for children who have visual impairment as well as those who need tactile stimulation.

## *Taste and smell*

Food and drink are obvious media for stimulation of taste and smell. Make sure you offer a varied and interesting selection. I have also found pot pourri very useful. As well as having an interesting smell, a child can get her hands in it for tactile stimulation. Aromatherapy oils such as lavender, camomile, (and from about 6 months old) mandarin, sandalwood, tea-tree and eucalyptus (very good for colds), orange, grapefruit, lemon, rose (for those who can afford it!), myrtle, geranium and ylang-ylang offer pleasing olfactory stimulation as well as having therapeutic benefits.

To stimulate taste buds you can offer your child a variety of small tastes of warm and cold things and sharp, sour, sweet etc. Examples are ice lollies, pieces of lemon, honey, tiny tastes of marmite, yoghurt etc.

# Involving your child in family life

Involve your child fully in family life. Let him help with chores if he is able. If he is not able, explain to him what you are doing. All children love making cakes. Even if mobility is severely affected he can still enjoy this activity with help. Children love to follow their parents around while they are doing the housework or the garden. If he can't do this, make sure he knows what you are doing and take some time to help him copy you. Children usually love watching television. I would recommend that a child who has CP should get the opportunity of the stimulation television can offer at least on a controlled basis, especially where the carer's time is severely restricted. It is better than leaving a child without any stimulation. A trip to the shops is interesting for a child even if it is a pain for the parent. There is a lot to be learned on the shelves in the supermarket.

If a child with disabilities is to have every opportunity to grow up with perceptions of the world which are similar to his non-disabled peers, full involvement with everyday activities is essential. Too much segregation and 'specialised' activity increase disadvantage by setting him further apart. Many 'so called' success stories of adults with CP occur where as children they lived in busy, active families in which they were treated as near to the same as everyone else as their disability allowed.

# 5

# Alternative and complementary treatments

There has been a general shift in attitude over recent years in regard to the use of alternative (or complementary as is now becoming the preferred term) treatments in this country. What used to be considered 'cranky' and 'off beat' is often now recognised to have a basis in fact. Many of the so-called alternative treatments available today have direct parallels in the more conventional medical system.

Treatments which have been used for centuries have been adopted by science but brought under a more controlled environment which can be clinically tested.

Herbalism is a good example of this trend. Many pharmaceutical drugs administered by doctors are chemical compounds which have been synthesised from the exact same ingredients found in the herbal remedy which can be used in its place.

Alternative medicine is no more able to cure cerebral palsy than conventional methods. However, there may be more gentle, enjoyable and even more effective ways to alleviate some of the effects of cerebral palsy and to cure (or avoid) many of the common illnesses which can cause so much more distress to a child who has CP.

The therapies outlined in this chapter are not an exhaustive list but they are the most commonly available forms of alternative treatment. Names and addresses of therapy centres and organisations which specialise in the various techniques can be found in the list of useful addresses and contacts on page 219.

Many alternative methods take a very different view of the diagnosis of a condition from that of mainstream Western medicine. Conventional medicine observes symptoms (problems which are presented and are directly observable) and seeks to alleviate the distress caused by symptoms or to eliminate the symptoms by suppressing them. The usual methods entail the use of drugs and/or surgery.

Alternative systems prefer to observe the 'whole person'. Symptoms are seen in the context of a person's overall physical and emotional health. They also attempt to examine and treat causes rather than symptoms. To do this alternative practitioners will take detailed histories of their patients and will seek to identify the central weakness which may be causing a chain reaction of ill health and which may well present as illness in another part of the body altogether.

It is essential with all forms of treatment, and alternative medicine is no exception, that you consult a practitioner in the field rather than administering for yourself out of lay persons' guides. Few of the following methods have been tried and tested under clinical conditions but many people who use alternative medicine have observed their positive effects. In addition, the negative side-effects of trying out alternative methods are far fewer than those often experienced under conventional medical treatment.

# Acupuncture

Acupuncture has been used as a conventional medicine in China for as long as records exist and is still a major treatment system often offered alongside Western techniques which have found their way into Chinese medicine. Diagnosis is carried out by measuring the energy flow in a number of meridians which form pathways (similar to a very fine nervous system) throughout the body. The energy levels are measured by taking pulses (of which the system identifies 27). The 10 internal organs (gallbladder, liver, lungs, colon, stomach, spleen, heart, small intestine, bladder and kidney) are perceived to carry the burden of any imbalance in the body. The vocabulary of acupuncture is very different from that of conventional medicine. The basic elements of water, wood, fire, earth and metal are considered to be reflected in the human body and an imbalance in these elements may be perceived as causal. There is also an emphasis on achieving a balance, in the body, of the opposite (but not antagonistic) qualities of yin and yang. Yin is cold, dark and feminine and yang is warm, light and masculine. A balance of both of these qualities is considered necessary for health. The energy flow which passes down the meridians is known as ch'i (pronounced 'chee'). Skin colour and body odour will also be noted and taken into account in diagnosis as well as a patient's fears, dislikes and preferences; for example, for seasons, drink and colours. The organs are considered to have a mother and child relationship and stimulation given to the mother organ will be expected to treat the child organ. For example the kidney/ bladder is mother to the liver/gallbladder and stimulation to the meridian of the kidney will automatically stimulate the liver.

Treatment is carried out by stimulating various points on the meridian which enable ch'i to flow more freely and affect the organ identified as causing problems. Stimulation will be in the form of acupuncture (using a fine needle which is partially inserted into the skin), acupressure (using finger tip pressure) or moxa (the application of heat). Many acupuncturists will supplement their treatment with Chinese herbs to be taken in between treatment sessions.

Many of the painful or distressing symptoms which occur as a result of having cerebral palsy may be lessened by acupuncture. Also, diagnosis by an acupuncturist may reveal conditions which have gone unnoticed by traditional methods.

Examples of treatable conditions may be: constipation, colic, high muscle tone (tight muscles), spasms, convulsions, depression, lethargy, poor concentration and sleeplessness.

It is possible that an acupuncturist may reveal an unexpected underlying cause for symptoms you present to him or her. My own experience demonstrates this. I took Danny to an acupuncturist with a view to getting treatment for his spasms and tightness of muscle. After taking a detailed history and examining Danny he informed me that Danny had had colic all of his life and that this was probably contributing not only to frequency of spasm and tightness of muscle but also to poor appetite, constipation and difficulty sleeping. He also said that Danny was extremely cold and gave him moxa treatment to counter this. After one treatment Danny's stomach was more relaxed than it had ever been before and his general tightness relaxed a little. I had always assumed that his tight muscles were purely the result of brain damage but, in fact, his upset digestive system was significantly contributing to the problem and this is treatable. His spasms increased initially but then settled down to a lesser level than prior to treatment.

# Homoeopathy

Homoeopathy is based on the principle that 'like cures like'. A minute dose of a preparation is administered which emulates the condition being treated in order to combat that condition. Homoeopaths believe in the body's ability to heal itself, and see symptoms as the body's way of striving to achieve that cure. The symptoms therefore, must reach an extreme peak in order for the body effectively to carry out its self-healing function. The role of the homoeopath is to find the homoeopathic drug which will enable the body to carry out this function. The current use of vaccinations under conventional medicine uses a similar principle to that of homoeopathy but without the detailed analysis which this school of medicine engages in.

During treatment symptoms are expected to worsen in the initial phase. Homoeopaths believe that symptoms are indications of the body's healing process and that the clue to treatment lies with the person. They will attempt to understand the person in terms of personality, current stresses in life, state of mind and preferences and dislikes in order to support the patient in battling against whatever condition is causing him discomfort. Over the past 175 years in excess of 2000 substances which produce certain symptoms have been developed by homoeopaths. These substances are minute and very diluted doses of animal, mineral or vegetable origin designed to encourage symptoms to work more effectively in the healing process. As with Chinese medicine the effects of weather, time of day, seasons, atmosphere and many other outside influences on the patient's symptoms will be considered. The quality of bodily excretion will be taken into account.

Many of the substances used in homoeopathy are poisonous if given in sufficient quantity but the quantity is the key to this form of treatment. Extremely diluted doses are often found to be the most effective. Homoeopathic remedies tend to be highly diluted for chronic conditions and diluted to a lower degree for acute conditions.

The homoeopath is committed to discovering the deepest and most individual remedy for each person, taking on board that person's unique symptoms and reactions to the environment as well as their moods and likes and dislikes.

Treatment is given in the form of small pills. Sometimes they are dissolvable. They taste of sugar and contain minute doses of the chosen homoeopathic remedy which has been diluted to the required level for the type of condition and the person being treated. Once administered, and if the remedy is working at its most effective, the symptoms being treated will probably intensify or get worse before they gradually disappear. Your homoeopath will be able to advise you regarding the length of time this process is likely to take. Some homoeopathic remedies are available in the form of ointment for treating skin conditions, stings and bruising etc. Some remedies are designed to offer instant relief in cases such as injury, shock and some other acute conditions.

# Herbalism

The use of herbs to treat illness has been available in most cultures throughout history. In Britain herbs fell from favour as conventional medicine began to take hold during the 18th century. However, the use of herbs has remained fairly commonplace although their medicinal properties are no longer recognised by the medical profession. I remember when I was working in a nursing home for elderly people being surprised to find that the elderly ladies knew all about the healing properties of comfrey which I had recently discovered. Comfrey is a traditional soother for rubbed skin and bruising. Occasionally, medical scientific investigations will prove the healing properties of a herbal preparation (as has happened recently with a Chinese herbal remedy for skin conditions). When this happens the research tends to focus on developing a chemical compound which will synthetically reproduce the same effect and which can then be mass produced by pharmaceutical companies. Chemical compounds are preferred by the medical profession because they are more easy to control, monitor and administer than their natural equivalents. Herbalists maintain that chemical compounds tend to have more severe side-effects than the natural herb. Natural herbs are more subtle in their immediate effect on the body and tend to diffuse more easily into the system which is therefore more able to accommodate the preparation. Chemical alternatives are often more severe and limited to the specific symptoms which a condition presents.

Herbalism, in a similar way to homoeopathy, aims to restore lost balance in the body by supporting the body's own 'self-righting' mechanisms. By administering the whole plant, rather than a specific derivative from a plant, a more wide ranging effect is achieved providing a general enhancing of resistance or of the functioning of a particular system in the body. Herbalists do not reject conventional medicine out of hand. Rather, they are likely to maintain that early treatment with gentle plant remedies when the first signs of poor health occur can often restore a healthy balance without the need for recourse to more drastic drug treatment. For example, antibiotics, used sparingly in serious situations (such as pneumonia) can be valuable and life-saving. However, if suitable plant remedies had been prescribed as soon as early symptoms of infection (raised temperature, catarrh etc.) were evident the infection would be very likely to have been arrested and resolved at a much earlier stage.

The remedies suggested below are suitable for everyone and may specifically be useful in common health problems affecting children who have cerebral palsy.

These herbs are all gentle in action and readily available. Most can be given as teas. The dose is not critical but two teaspoons of dried herb per cup is a standard rough guide for adults. This should be halved for children and halved again for small babies. Teas are made by adding boiling water to the herb and allowing it to stand (covered so that volatile oils are not lost in evaporation) for 5–10 minutes. Then strain and sweeten, if desired, with apple concentrate or honey. Give three or four times daily.

## Respiratory infections

Colds, coughs, catarrh, sore throat etc.:

- **Sage** – particularly good as a gargle or drunk slowly for sore throats;
- **Thyme** – too strong for very young children but useful added to sage for sore throats and minor chest infections (using half the usual dose);
- **Elderflower** – excellent for upper respiratory catarrh, induces sweating and sleep;
- **Yarrow** – another good remedy for stimulating elimination by sweating;
- **Hyssop** – useful for chest infections and chronic catarrh (an expectorant);
- **Elecampane** – very good for chest infections and for use as an expectorant; the root is used so a decoction has to be made – add cold water to the shredded root and allow to stand overnight before bringing to the boil;

- **Garlic** – marvellous for preventing and curing infection. Chop up the cloves finely and add them to honey so that the mixture may be swallowed without chewing. One or two teaspoons of the mixture should be given at bed time. Fresh lemon juice may be added to the mixture. Garlic is powerfully bactericidal and is excreted via the lungs (hence the smell on the breath) so is particularly appropriate for chest infections. It sounds dreadful but actually doesn't taste that bad. Many children will take this mixture without protest.

## Sleeplessness and nervous excitability

Gentle calming herbs include **chamomile, lemon balm, lime flowers** and **lavender**.

The first three make excellent teas and the last is probably best used as an oil added to bath water at bed time. It is also worth trying these gentle herbs if your child is having lots of fits. There are other herbs traditionally used for treating fits but a qualified herbalist should be consulted before these are considered.

## Constipation

Diet is probably the most important factor here and the addition of prunes, and cold-pressed olive oil or sunflower oil to food should help.

A safe remedy which may help is linseed or psyllium seed. Soak a teaspoon of the seeds in a cup of hot water for two hours then drink the tea and eat the seeds (this might be difficult for a child who finds it difficult to swallow solids). The seeds swell up and the bulking action should stimulate the bowel.

This remedy needs to be taken for a week or two (once a day) before the effect is established.

See also the recipe for relief of constipation given on page 38.

# Osteopathy and cranial osteopathy

In common with other alternative practitioners, osteopaths believe that their treatment should seek to enable the body's own healing mechanisms to correct any imbalance which has developed and which is causing pain, discomfort or illness.

Osteopathy is particularly appropriate for treating conditions which arise as a result of muscular or skeletal dysfunction.

Dysfunction is seen to arise and to worsen as a result of the brain's response to muscular or skeletal tension or alignment.

The brain is constantly monitoring every muscle and joint and is accustomed to a set of norms for muscular tension and the position of joints. If a joint (for example, a vertebra) jolts out of alignment due to an accident or for any other reason a flood of impulses report the injury to the brain. Muscles which support the spine will tense up to protect the area and the brain re-assesses 'normal' and tries to accommodate the body's new state. As a result, after the injury has healed the tension in the surrounding muscles may remain thereby rendering the joint susceptible to further injury or permanently out of line and unable to return to the normal, relaxed state.

Osteopathy works at ways to allow the body to reset its own norms which are then translated to the brain so that the original state of equilibrium is restored. At its most extreme this is achieved by the osteopath delivering small movements with high force onto the specific problem area/joint with the intention of sending a more appropriate set of impulses through the muscular system and message to the brain.

Cranial osteopathy is more complex than conventional osteopathy. It works on the principle that the body contains a number of basic rhythms (for example breathing, circulation, primary respiratory movement in all of the body's tissues and cranial sacrum rhythm). The whole body flexes and extends slightly in its natural state and these movements are reflected in the movement of the cranium. The cranium is the bone structure which surrounds the brain and which interlocks but also has flexibility which enables flexion and extension to take place within the skull area up to 6–10 times per minute. These movements can react upon movement in the brain, spinal cord, sacrum and limbs. Underlying cranial osteopathy is the notion that we develop patterns during our lives which may cause restriction in the natural flow of flexion and extension. Cranial osteopaths set out to correct any imbalance by enabling the cranial area to recover its natural flow.

Osteopathy cannot cure the brain damage which causes cerebral palsy. It is possible, however, that a number of the incorrect patterns of muscular tension and skeletal position which result from the brain damage send back further incorrect messages to the brain which further exacerbate the negative effects of the muscular and skeletal system. It is possible that osteopathy, gently and sensitively applied, may be able to avert a chain reaction which often creates more extreme tension and bone deformity than the original brain damage warrants.

# Reflexology

The main principle of reflexology is that there is a direct reflex action between the nerve endings in the feet and various organs in the body. Light pressure applied to the appropriate nerve ending in the foot which correlates to an affected organ is said to bring relief to the condition caused by that particular organ dysfunction. This system can be used to diagnose, prevent and treat disorders. The reflexologist holds the patient's feet and uses sensitive fingers to read the surface. During treatment a stable pressure is maintained on the appropriate point of the foot while a clockwise rotating movement of the hand is applied continuously.

Reflexology is one of the few alternative techniques which has been tested with patients who have CP. Many patients have reported that pain and spasm decreased.

Reflexology is thought to be particularly useful in the treatment of congestion, constipation, dispersal of toxins in the body and improvement of energy flow.

# Aromatherapy

Aromatherapy is an ancient healing technique based on the use of aromatic essential oils and essences extracted from flowers, plants, resins and other substances. The treatment is absorbed through the skin (the body's largest organ) and passes very quickly into the bloodstream. Treatment is applied through gentle massage. The physical benefits of massage for people who have CP can be wide ranging. It stimulates the circulation of blood and lymph (which deals with toxins in the body), stimulates the immune system, reduces muscular tension and reduces pain in muscles and joints. A good massage can be as refreshing and relaxing as sleep, especially since muscles often remain tense even in sleep.

Certain oils have chemical constituents in them which will affect the brain and have a sedating or anti-depressant effect. Many of the common problems associated with CP may be helped with aromatherapy. For example, there are oils which work against chest infection (expectorant oils which shift and loosen mucus) so it will be possible for the child to cough them up. These oils can be burnt in the room for long periods of time to keep the benefits building up. A daily stomach massage (in a clockwise direction) is one of the best ways to shift faeces around the intestines to combat constipation. Certain oils used in combination with the massage will increase its effectiveness. There are certain oils which stimulate the immune system and help children to fight off infections; some may even prevent infections if used regularly.

Research scientists have tested aromatherapy oils and found that there are indeed chemical properties which can be recognised within the oils and which are of therapeutic benefit for certain disorders.

Almost all paramedics will agree that the stimulation offered by massage and by aromatic oils is in itself beneficial. This is especially so where a child has sensory impairment, as both touch and smell are being encouraged to develop.

## Other alternative treatments

There are very many more alternative or complementary systems available. It is not possible to detail them all but the following might also be of interest:

### Alexander technique

This form of re-education is used primarily to get rid of faulty habits such as bad posture, over-tension, incorrect breathing and speech defects.

### Kinesiology

Kinesiology is the science of muscle testing to determine the interrelationship of the physiological processes in the body with respect to movement. It is thought that kinesiology may be able to detect energy imbalance before many other tests.

### Shiatsu massage

Shiatsu involves the correction of faulty circulation, improvement of metabolism and treatment of a number of ailments by massage to meridia connecting points just beneath the surface of the skin.

## Spiritual healing

Spiritual healing is concerned with the transfer of energy from healer to patient. This energy is known as 'prana' or universal life force for which the healer acts as a channel.

## Yoga

This self-help exercise and meditation system can help to reduce stress and relieve muscle tension, as well as contributing to all round fitness.

# 6

# Informal support, social factors and disadvantage

## The home environment

A human being's basic needs are for food, rest, warmth and shelter. In addition to these are a host of emotional and intellectual needs which are necessarily met by direct interaction with others be it spoken, felt, or seen and heard as through reading or music. Most of us take the basic needs totally for granted, but many people with disabilities cannot. Severity of disability will affect the extent to which a disabled person is dependent on others, but there are often ways of reducing the dependence.

There are basically two issues which should be considered in giving a person with disabilities full opportunity to independence in the home. These are:

- The housing design;
- Help within the home to live life independently.

The way in which your accommodation is designed can make a significant contribution towards your independence in the home. Architects and providers of housing are beginning to realise the importance of accessible design for people with disabilities.

### Housing design

The two main types of self-contained dwelling construction for people with disabilities are mobility housing and wheelchair housing. For those who need extra support, shared housing (sometimes with a live-in warden) is a possibility.

**Mobility housing**  This is built to normal space standards but includes features such as ramped entrance, wide doors, mechanical access to upper room (either by lift or stair lift) and bedrooms and bathrooms on the ground floor. These standards are designed to meet the needs of people who can walk a little but who may need to use a wheelchair some of the time.

**Wheelchair housing**   This is designed specially for people who are permanently confined to a wheelchair or use a wheelchair most of the time. Special consideration will be given to the ground level on approach to the property, internal planning to allow a wheelchair to manoeuvre, doorways of a width to ensure easy passage of a wheelchair, kitchen and bathroom planning to allow for use from a wheelchair, switches and door and window handles placed appropriately for operation from a wheelchair.

Under the provisions of The Chronically Sick and Disabled Persons Act 1970, local authorities are required to consider housing needs in their areas in respect of registered disabled people. These responsibilities are interpreted very differently from authority to authority.

**The British Standards Institute Codes of Practice**   Design of housing for the convenience of disabled people provides a standard that, whenever practicable, ordinary housing should be convenient for disabled occupants or visitors. There are a number of other British Standard codes available from The British Standards Institute (see the list of contacts and useful addresses on page 219).

Considerations in design include the following:

- Doorways and hallways should be wide enough for wheelchairs;
- Ramps should be used instead of steps;
- Stair lifts should be installed where steps are unavoidable;
- Sinks, cookers and other kitchen appliances should be within easy reach with handles that are easy to operate;
- Windows should be easy to open;
- Plugs, switches and sockets need to be within easy reach;
- Easy access to gardens is important;
- Space standards in bathrooms must allow for wheelchair access;

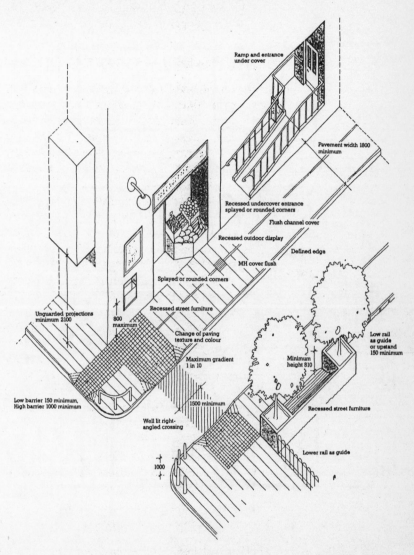

*Good housing design: access (courtesy of Islington Council).*

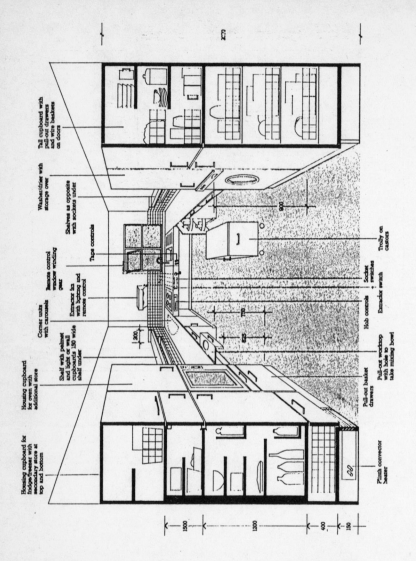

*Good housing design: kitchens (courtesy of Islington Council).*

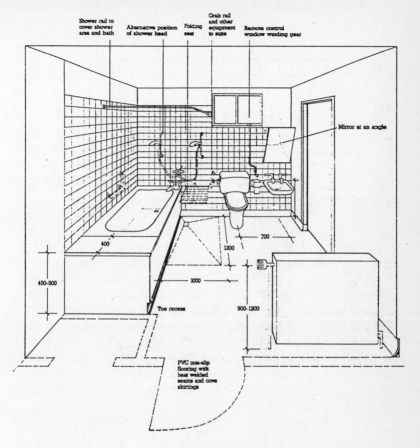

Shower rail to cover shower area and bath · Alternative position of shower head · Folding seat · Grab rail and other equipment to suite · Remote control window winding gear

Mirror at an angle

400

450-500

700

1200

1000

Toe recess

900-1200

PVC non-slip flooring with heat welded seams and cove skirtings

*Good housing design: bathrooms (courtesy of Islington Council).*

- Hoists may be needed to help with bathing and getting the disabled person in and out of bed;
- Heating should be adequate and easily controlled;
- Good insulation should be installed;
- Toilets may need to be adapted so that the user can be independent if at all possible.

If your home needs adaptations, or if you feel you need to relocate to another house in order to have a properly accessible home, your first point of contact will probably be the local Housing Department. Some Housing Departments employ access officers who specialise in accessible design. Another good source of support is Housing Associations, especially those who specialise in housing people with disabilities (see the list of contacts and useful addresses on pages 219–231). An occupational therapist will normally become involved in helping to organise the home for maximum independence.

There are a number of organisations who can offer advice on adaptations to the home, as well as on equipment which can be installed in the home to facilitate independent living. The Disabled Living Foundation keep a comprehensive collection of aids and appliances, equipment and design criteria which can be viewed by appointment. There are also a number of touring aids exhibitions including the Mobile Aids Centre and the RADAR Travelling Aids Exhibition (see the list of useful addresses and contacts on page 219).

## *Owner occupiers and private tenants*

You may be entitled to a Housing Renovation Grant intended to allow for upgrading properties built before October 1961 (in practice this cut off date is flexible depending on individual need). To qualify you must be a freeholder, leaseholder or a regulated or secure tenant. The local authority will not provide the entire cost but a fixed percentage. In some cases Social Services may be able to help you bear the remainder. Advice should be sought from your local Social Services Department.

Home Improvement Grants may be available by application to the local authority. These are intended to help bring homes up to a good standard.

Repair Grants may be available if your house needs structural repairs and was built before 1919.

# Local authority tenants

If you live in a council house which requires adaptation you should apply to the housing office in the first instance. It will usually be necessary to involve an occupational therapist to assess your adaptation needs and report to the local authority. Once this has been done, the local authority may pay for all or part of the adaptation necessary. Some local authorities have a number of new units which are built to mobility or wheelchair standard but this provision varies greatly across the country.

A number of local authorities have produced their own guidelines for design standards to be adhered to when providing housing for people with disabilities. Where these guidelines exist they will be available from the local authority's surveyors' or architects' department.

# Housing Associations (HAs)

Housing Associations are specialised housing organisations which are partly funded by Central Government and partly funded by private finance. HA tenants do not have security of tenure although they do have some security under a tenants' guarantee.

Housing Associations have a reputation for the high standards of conversion and new building work that they often produce. There are a number of Housing Associations which specialise either exclusively or partially in providing housing to meet the needs of people with disabilities (see the list of useful addresses and contacts, on pages 219–231). Housing Association rents can sometimes (but not always) be considerably higher than those set by local authorities.

Some Housing Associations specialise in shared housing which basically entails the provision of group homes in which a number of people with physical or mental disabilities share certain amenities (such as kitchens and bathrooms) but have their own rooms as well. If residents require a high level of support, shared houses will often have a flat provided within them to house a warden.

## Housing co-operatives

There are three main types of housing co-operative:

- Those which operate similarly to Housing Associations in terms of the type of dwelling produced and source of finance (these are called par value co-operatives);
- Tenant management co-operatives – groups of tenants of local authorities or Housing Associations who band together to form a group who manage their own homes collectively;
- Private finance co-operatives, consisting of groups of people who get together to raise private mortgages to develop their homes collectively.

The way in which co-operative housing differs from other kinds of housing provision is that those who live in co-operative homes also control the way in which the housing is managed. Par value and private finance co-ops also control the way in which their housing is developed. This means that individual tenants can have a large say in the way their homes are designed and in the way the housing is managed (in terms of maintenance etc.) once they are occupied.

Co-operative housing could offer an ideal opportunity to people with disabilities in that they could be fully involved in consultation about the design of their homes in the early stages. Sadly, housing co-operatives have a very poor record in the area of housing provision for the disabled. Awareness is growing and a number of co-operatives are now taking the initiative to ensure that people with disabilities get an opportunity to join. However, in many cases co-ops rely on the local authority to refer people with disabilities and these referrals often come too late for the disabled person to enjoy the consultation opportunities open to other co-op members.

You should be able to get a list of Tenant Management Co-ops from your local Housing Department and a list of par value co-operatives from the Housing Corporation or the National Federation of Housing Associations.

## Support in the home: statutory services

**Home helps** Social services can provide domestic and other help (such as help with shopping) through the home help service. The service is not sufficient to provide full independence to a severely disabled person but can be a useful back-up to other services.

**Laundry service** A laundry service can be provided by Social Services but there may be a charge depending on the family's income.

**Meals on wheels** Volunteers deliver meals to your home organised by the local authority. There may be a charge for the service.

**District nurses** The Health Authority employ trained nurses to pay regular visits to provide domestic health care such as help getting in and out of bed and bathing. Referrals are usually through your GP.

## Community Service Volunteers (CSV)

Under the Independent Living Project, CSV can provide volunteers who contract to work for a number of months providing the level of assistance required for independent living. In some cases this might include a 24 hour service entailing 2–3 volunteers working in shifts. The local Social Services will sometimes support these schemes with supervision for volunteers and funding.

## Centres for independent living

**SHAD (Sheltered Housing Assistance for the Disabled)** SHAD was established to enable severely disabled people to live in their own homes and lead independent lives in the community.

**Derbyshire Independent Living Project** Developed by the Derbyshire coalition of disabled people, this centre is modelled on the centres for independent living which operate in the United States. The prime objective is to provide care attendants to facilitate independent living.

**Hampshire Centre for Independent Living** This was designed to help severely disabled people to find alternative accommodation and support outside residential care. The centre seeks to advance the education of the public regarding the needs and potential of people with disabilities.

**BCODP (British Council of Organisations of Disabled People)**   BCODP believes that every disabled person has a right to make his or her own decision regarding the preferred form of housing. BCODP is keen to promote the involvement of people with disabilities in the development of their housing from a very early stage.

**The Centre on Environment for the Handicapped**   This centre provides a specialist information and advisory service on the environmental needs of people with disabilities. It also holds a register of housing and care support schemes.

**RADAR (Royal Association for Disability and Rehabilitation)**   RADAR has a housing department which offers advice and guidance. This undertakes research into the housing needs of people with disabilities and pressures local authorities to improve provision.

**Shelter**   Shelter is a charity which helps homeless people and has been particularly interested in provision for people with disabilities and community care initiatives since The Year of the Disabled (1981).

**Scope**   This society works to estabish independent living opportunities in various parts of the country, often in association with Housing Associations.

## Residential accommodation

The inability of families to maintain adequate provision of care has been found to be the major precipitating factor leading to a person with disabilities entering residential accommodation, the most common problems being parental ill health or death. Traditionally residential care has tended to be medically based with the disabled resident being expected to assume the role of 'sick' person. Times are slowly changing and there is a move amongst providers of residential settings to try to develop more along the group homes line, providing people with disabilities with as much independence as is possible. Unfortunately, however, large numbers of traditional residential units do still exist where residents (whether or not they will it) live in a state of total dependence on staff.

Scope runs a number of residential homes and is taking an active role in the move towards a more independent orientation for those who have been living in institutionalised settings. The prime objectives of Scope's residential policy are:

- That every person with cerebral palsy has the right to self-determination;
- That every person with cerebral palsy should have the option of having his own accommodation;
- That every person with cerebral palsy should be assisted to use community facilities if he chooses to do so;
- That every person with cerebral palsy should be given the opportunity to learn new skills;
- That the key investment of service provision should not be in large, institutional buildings, but in people providing appropriate assistance;
- That every person with cerebral palsy has the right to share equally in the benefits and difficulties of life in the community and should be encouraged to participate in the mainstream of community life as much as possible.

Scope offers a service of Individual Programme Plans by which a person with cerebral palsy is assisted to develop a plan of action regarding their future, setting goals and making plans to achieve them. Everyone who is in this scheme will have an advocate who is someone able to support them and represent them in pursuing their own plan.

## Camphill residential communities

Inspired by the teaching and philosophy of Rudolph Steiner, the Camphill Communities aim to provide a creative, nurturing and secure environment tailored to meet the individual needs of each resident. The staff have a one-to-one ratio to residents and live alongside residents participating equally with them in community life.

Basic to the philosophy of Camphill is the unique and positive contribution that each individual makes. The organisation believes that every individual is educable, and that there is useful and rewarding work that every individual can participate in.

Camphill Communities exist, usually in the country, to serve the needs of physically and mentally disabled people who are not able to live at home with their families or independently in the community. They run communities which are specifically for:

- Children;
- Adults with severe disabilities;
- Adults with less severe disabilities, needing less intensive support.

The teaching within the community includes a great emphasis on the creative arts which are utilised to help residents to realise their own potential. People with different disabilities are integrated within the community on the principle that this provides for fuller integration and mutual support.

For more information see the list of useful addresses and contacts on page 219.

## Friends and family

This section considers the positive and negative reactions that the parents and carers of children with cerebral palsy may encounter among their friends and other family members, and considers ways of utilising or coping with them.

### Friends

A number of mothers have talked to me of the loneliness they experienced following the birth of their children. This can happen whether or not your child has a disability but, for mothers whose children do have disabilities, the isolation is accentuated by many factors.

I am particularly stressing the position of mothers here because they are often the ones who carry the weight of the family, especially in the early days. In addition to being the person who makes the closest contact with the child in the earliest days, mothers have to cope with physical weakness, possible post-natal depression, catering for other members of the family and somehow finding some space for themselves in amongst all of this.

Friends may be fearful that your needs as a mother will be beyond the scope of what they feel able to give. Often they will avoid you rather than talking to you about your situation. Friends who have the best intentions in the world are not immune from society's negative images of disability. They may feel afraid of disability, unable to know how to communicate and tend to steer clear of the situation rather than face it. The first they may hear is that there is something 'wrong' with your child, probably well before they actually see you again following the birth or diagnosis. This will allow plenty of time for wild imaginations to run riot from the starting point of *'wrong'*. On the other hand friends can be your best source of strength in those early days when you are adjusting. Friends may really want to support you and share your experiences but they may need your guidance on how to go about it. The best way to get support from your friends is to ask for specific things which are quantifiable in both time and effort. If your friends know exactly where they stand and what is required of them they will be more likely to enjoy the experience and less afraid of it. Perhaps you can start by inviting them round for an informal meal and getting them to hold and play with your child while you prepare the food. Once they are used to the child (and he is used to them) they may be happy to progress on to short spells of babysitting.

## Fathers

In the early days, if you have a partner, he too, like friends, can be a source of strength. When two parents are involved there is real opportunity to share anxieties, work out strategies for dealing with problems and share the joys of each small success. On the other hand, many fathers quickly become exasperated with the sudden loss of attention from their partner and resent the intrusion of the child. Again, this can apply whether or not your child is disabled. There is an intense learning process which inevitably takes place around having a child who has disabilities and this increases the likelihood that the father will feel pushed out. Mothers often tend to bond more quickly with children and may find it easier than fathers to make contact with their child. Fathers may experience their child's disability in a much more negative way. This is hardly surprising in a world where there are constant images of 'perfection' which we are all meant to strive for and which men are expected to uphold and procreate. The sense of failure can be overwhelming for a father. There are proportionately more families with a disabled member that are single parent families than those without. My advice to mothers is that you involve your partner fully in every aspect of your child's development. Even if he is out at work all day and misses the hours you might spend in waiting rooms at doctors' and therapists' surgeries you can discuss this with him and involve him in any decision making. Try to make sure he gets an opportunity to develop a relationship with the child while he is at home. You might find that you instinctively want to dominate his interaction with your child as it is you who are receiving direct advice on how best to cater for her needs. However, it might be better for Dad just to get to know his child even if it does mean that he is holding her the wrong way! To be fair to fathers I must add that I have met some great dads who really participate in their children's upbringing and take a fair share in the care and development as well as decision making about their children.

## Siblings

Brothers and sisters play a very important role in the life of a child who has disabilities and vice versa. There are two distinct ways this can develop with a variety of overlap in between. An older brother or sister can be a protective and caring friend to the young sibling. On the other hand the older child may experience jealousy and isolation when a lot of energy and attention appear to be concentrated on a sibling who might not even seem to respond very much. However, children often expect less from others anyway. I have seen many a situation where the disability of another child doesn't even register while the parent of the non-disabled child is plainly uncomfortable. We can learn a lot from children in this respect. I have seen older brothers and sisters quite happily interacting with their younger brothers and sisters who have disabilities without even considering that they are in any way 'different'.

Make the most of every opportunity to involve older children in your child's life and development. Take the risk of letting them cart the little one around and play with him, even if it looks a bit dangerous. As long as you are on hand to rescue the situation it can only help to cement a bond between siblings and provide your child with disabilities with vital and interesting stimulation. Over-protection is probably one of the worst disservices you can do to a child who has disabilities. He is just a kid like any other and he needs to get a chance to experience that. My own eldest son, Tam, went through a year of jealousy and very real trauma while trying to remake his place in my life against the seemingly endless demands of his little brother. Eventually, he began to appreciate that he had a smaller person in his life that he could dominate, be a role model for, gain admiration from and share with. Now they like to cuddle up together to watch cartoons on the television on a Saturday morning but it was a long haul to get to that. It is very important that you do not let your older children get to a stage when they feel neglected. This is a common experience regardless of the existence of disability. Older children need to feel that they are still loved and valued. Trusting them with your smaller child is one way to do this. Another way is to ensure that the older child gets a special time for him, even if it means leaving your younger child to fend for himself a little occasionally. The experience will probably do the younger child the world of good.

Siblings that are younger can be a source of inspiration to your older child as well as to you. As they grow they can also become role models for your child who has disabilities. The older child can also gain a sense of power (a very difficult thing to do if you are disabled) if they have a younger sibling to contend with.

There are a number of entertaining children's books which are intended to promote positive images of children who have disabilities (see the further reading list on page 232). Introducing these books to siblings may help them to feel proud of their brother or sister who has a disability and to understand that the individual is more important than the disability.

## Extra problems encountered by single parents

An enormous burden is placed on the single parent. Not only do you have the job of nurturing your child and facilitating her development, but you are also responsible for bringing in the financial resources to enable the family to survive. Being a single parent is challenge enough by itself without the extra responsibility of bringing up a child who has disabilities which need to be confronted. Extra help is available to single parents; unfortunately you may have to go out and seek it but it *is* there if you know where to go. Voluntary groups, parent support groups and Social Services should be at your disposal. Make sure that you use whatever facilities are available in your area. You can start with Scope. They now have a Helpline for carers and people with CP (see the list of useful addresses and contacts on page 219). A sympathetic social worker can put you in touch with all kinds of voluntary and statutory assistance.

## Extra problems encountered by families with more than one disabled member

Twin births which have complications or are premature run a higher risk of one or both children developing cerebral palsy. If both are affected it is unlikely that it will be to the same degree. Also, having one child with a disability is no guarantee that subsequent children will not be disabled (although it is statistically unlikely).

Each individual responds differently to their circumstances. The problems experienced by the parents of more than one disabled child will be similar to those of carers of one child with a disability but the issues will all become intensified. Coping ability is likely to be stretched to the limit and the psychological trauma more severe. Transport can be more difficult to arrange. The possibility of becoming isolated and housebound increases. Financial problems are likely to be severe. On top of this there will be a double schedule of treatment/therapy to accommodate.

It is especially important for carers of more than one child who have disabilities to get access to relief and support. Respite care, home help, help with care in the home, benefits and grants should all be utilised (see Chapter 9 on rights and benefits). You should ensure that you are referred to a social worker who can channel every available means of support to you – ask your GP or health visitor about this.

## Child abuse

Studies have suggested that up to 50 per cent of deaf children have experienced abuse. It has also been shown that the number decreases when the child is taught to sign and thereby given early communication. A disproportionate number of children with disabilities is likely to be victims of some form of abuse (the two main forms of child abuse are those involving violence and sex). The highest levels of abuse have been found to take place in residential homes. However, there is a higher than average level of abuse within the parental home as well.

The dividing line between discipline and violence may seem thin at times. If you are a parent of a child who has problems communicating, and maybe cries a lot as a result of her frustration, you may find it difficult to restrain yourself from hitting out at her – especially if you are worn out with sleepless nights and prolonged crying. The fact is, however, that children with limited mobility or who lack a means to communicate effectively are extremely vulnerable. They are in even less of a position than their non-disabled peers to hit back, shout out or run away. If you feel like hitting your child it would be kinder to leave the room even if it does mean leaving her on her own screaming her head off. If you need to get your aggression out – hit a pillow – *hard.* If you fear that you are unable to contain yourself there are helplines you can ring. Scope Cerebral Palsy Helpline is geared to give support in this area, as are Parents Anonymous and CRY-SIS. Pick up that phone before you hit out at your child. (See the list of useful addresses on pages 219–231 for more information.)

As with physical violence, sexual abuse of children with disabilities may be more common because of the child's inability to report what is happening to her. Non-disabled children who are abused often fail to report what is happening because they are afraid of losing the only security they know or because they are afraid of reprisals. If you suspect that your child, or a child you know, might be a victim of abuse you should contact Childline (See the list of useful addresses and contacts on page 219) for advice.

## Outside the home
### *Child care*

Getting decent child care is a problem for carers who wish or need to work when their children are small. Even as they grow older, school hours do not fit in with most working hours. Facilities which are sometimes available on school premises for after school care are less likely to be available for children who have disabilities. In addition, you will probably want a quality of care which ensures that your child's special needs are being catered for adequately while you are at work. Specially trained nannies are hard to come by and expensive. Au pairs are unlikely to have training (although enthusiasm can go a long way) and you need the extra space to house them as well as money to pay them. Childminders can be a good option but you will need to satisfy yourself that the childminder you choose is keen to facilitate your child's development. Nurseries may offer priority to children who have disabilities but, again, you need to be satisfied that they are geared up to meet your child's needs. Catering for your child's needs in a group setting does not necessarily mean that your child must be provided with special toys, particular attention or physical therapy. Attitude is just as important as all of these. A good childminder or nursery worker will be able to integrate your child by encouraging non-disabled peers to lose sight of any sense of 'difference' that they perceive in your child.

In some areas there are nurseries and under-fives facilities which cater specifically for children with disabilities but their existence does not guarantee you a place or that your child will be cared for according to your wishes. Seek advice from your local authority or Social Services. Your local branch of Scope may be able to offer advice.

Whatever form of child care you choose you will need to ensure that the people caring for your child are keen, interested and positive in their approach. You will also need to make sure that they are well acquainted with your child's particular needs, interests and method of communication.

## Everyday life out in the community

Your everyday life is affected by a great many factors. Family, friends, education, where you live, who you socialise with, your beliefs, your financial position, your employment situation, the amount of free time you have to yourself, your independence (physical or emotional) all play their part. For this reason it is not possible for any guide book to give advice which applies to everyone on participation in the community. There are some generalisations, however, which might apply to most people who have disabilities. Parents of children who have visible disabilities may feel embarrassed about these and tend to shy away from taking their children out in public. Attitudes are changing slowly but this continues to be an issue for many parents. If the reason is not embarrassment, the sheer difficulty of getting around might put parents off taking their children out and about. A vicious circle then emerges in which people with visible disabilities are viewed with suspicion and fear because so few of them get out into the world. This in turn contributes to embarrassment or fear on the part of parents, or even the person herself. Another common occurrence is the misplaced sympathetic gesture: strangers coming up and offering you or your child money, for example saying 'aah, the poor little thing'.

There are no easy ways of combating unwanted attitudes from the public. It is certain, though, that hiding children who have disabilities away at home will only serve to perpetuate misguided and negative images. If people with disabilities were more visible and active in the community we would eventually see a breaking down of the barriers.

It is often the way that, where discrimination exists, it is the people who suffer the discrimination who make the first move towards creating a shift in public opinion. Parent support groups can be helpful too. Parents working together with disabled adults are able to form pressure groups and lobby for changes in the environment such as ramps and disabled toilets in public places, to make access to the community easier or improve integration in mainstream playgroups and schools. Schools themselves can help by putting on shows and events which include positive images around disability. The same considerations should apply to the design of public buildings as in the organisation or adaptation of the home.

## Race, class and disability

Middle class, articulate, white parents are well placed to tap into services which are available for children who have disabilities. On the other hand black parents and parents who are less articulate may not even get into the system let alone reap any benefits from it.

Parents often have to 'discover for themselves' what their entitlements are to services and benefits. Those parents who are used to bureaucracy, or even have perhaps worked within the system, are bound to find the process of discovery easier than those whose cultural or class background differs.

Professionals have said to me, 'The resources are there for everyone but "they" don't come forward'. The onus often gets placed on the person who is having difficulties with the system in the first place to 'make the effort'. There may be many reasons why people do not come forward to take advantage of services. Professionals can go a long way towards redressing these imbalances by making the effort themselves to ensure that they explain to clients precisely what they are able to offer in language that is easy to understand. Physiotherapists and doctors, for example, should avoid using jargon and should clearly explain the purpose of certain exercises and treatments etc. Social workers and health visitors need to ensure that clients are aware of the statutory services and benefits to which they are entitled. It would help enormously if professionals such as health visitors could carry application forms for standard benefits around with them to hand out to clients. There should also be someone in Health Service employment who ensures that clients are put in touch with local and national voluntary agencies and charities who can offer support. Information sheets and leaflets should be translated into languages which are commonly used by local ethnic groups.

An even more complex issue than access to information and services is that of expectations and attitudes held by professionals. Racial discrimination and discrimination against people with disabilities have some parallels. Traditionally black people have been expected to integrate into British society and to turn their backs on their own systems and cultures. This is bound to lead to failure. You cannot expect a person to become someone different, and the attempt to force such changes on people from other cultures negates them and threatens the loss of the wealth of new experience which can be offered to the host culture. Similarly, people with disabilities are expected to strive to forsake their differences and to refashion themselves into a non-disabled mould. Not only is this impossible but it negates the positive contribution that a person with disabilities, just as she is, can make to society. Professionals and non-disabled people need to see the person first. Legislation can help to guard against overt discrimination in society but only willingness and effort from members of society who do not experience disadvantage is going to change the more covert discrimination expressed in negative attitudes and dismissal of the worth of people who are perceived as 'different'.

A person who is black and disabled is up against double discrimination. He may experience isolation in groups of white, disabled people or in groups of black, non-disabled people. He will be especially likely, therefore, to come up against prejudice. Publications addressing this issue are beginning to be produced and pressure groups are forming – see the list of useful addresses and contacts on pages 219–231.

## Gay and disabled

Discrimination against gays and lesbians may operate in a slightly different way in that sexual orientation is not generally visible. It depends on you whether or not you wish to be known as gay or lesbian. However, an enormous amount of prejudice exists against gays and lesbians. If you are disabled and open about your sexuality there may be a fear that you are more vulnerable to abuse or attack than a non-disabled gay person.

If you want to enjoy meeting others in the gay community and your mobility is restricted your choice about being open about your sexuality may be limited. It's a bit difficult for a gay person to get a parent to phone Dial-a-ride to enable him to attend a gay function without being open about his sexual preference.

There are no easy answers to these problems but supportive family and friends are essential for gay and lesbian people who have disabilities to enable them to enjoy a full life and have access to the lifestyle of their choice. Gay Switchboard may be able to offer some advice (see the list of contacts and useful addresses on page 219).

## Local, informal support groups

There will be some self-help support groups in most areas. Your local branch of Scope and the town hall should have a list of the local groups.

Support groups can work in a number of ways. Groups of parents who get together and identify common needs can often prove to be a powerful force in campaigning for improved services, introducing new ideas into a community and even setting up resource centres themselves.

Some groups may provide opportunities for parents to meet and discuss feelings and needs. A particularly successful support group in North London (the North London CD family support group) centres its activities on a regularly published, very informative newsletter which enables carers who cannot get out to meetings to benefit from the experiences of others in a similar situation.

Other groups might form with the specific purpose of increasing services to children via self-help (under parental control). In Islington, a group of parents has come together to start a play and learn group for children with disabilities. We have called the group PALACE (Play and Learn and Creative Education) and our aim is to prepare our children to enter mainstream education, give them opportunities for social integration and interaction with non-disabled children and complement local authority therapy with input from a Peto trained physiotherapist. We also involve volunteers in playing with our children while parents get together for discussions. This gives parents a break, allows children to build up relationships outside the family and offers valuable experience to the volunteers. Another group of Islington parents (whose children have recently left school with nowhere to go) have come together to create a facility for their children (based at a local community centre) which aims to create individual programmes for the young adults involved so that they can continue to develop and enjoy a social life in the community.

Groups such as these are being or have been set up in many parts of the country but finding out about them isn't always easy. Local branches of the larger disability organisations (such as Scope) may be able to help. The health professionals who come to see your child will often have heard of local groups.

## Fund raising

Resources cost money and not all will be available through social or educational services. While some argue that needs should all be met by statutory services, the hard facts are that not all necessarily will. However, if you come across equipment or treatment that you feel would be of benefit to your child it is wise to find out whether funding can be made available from the local authority before you embark on a strenuous fund raising exercise. Examples of the things for which you might wish to raise funds include the following:

- Therapy treatments which are not generally available in this country or not contained within the health service (such as patterning and conductive education);
- Setting up or running costs for support groups and self-help groups;
- Equipment such as computers, non-standard seating, video cameras (to facilitate progress monitoring), non-standard wheelchairs and walking frames, seating and buggies, adapted toys and learning aids.

I must stress that there is a lobby in the Disability Rights Movement which strongly objects to fund raising by donation (particularly the recently popular television events). There are a number of sound reasons for these objections:

- Reliance on charity detracts from the fact that people with disabilities have a right to services and equipment which meet their needs to enable them to participate equally in society;
- It perpetuates the idea that people with disabilities are somehow inadequate;
- It encourages people to sympathise and contribute due to guilt rather than to recognise the equal worth of people with disabilities;
- Giving donations may lead people to believe that they have in some way 'discharged their duty' where disability is concerned;
- With charitable funding the distribution of resources becomes very uneven. Only those projects and individuals who 'know the system' are likely to get access to charity;
- There is still not enough money available through these sources to really meet need.

The real need is for a change in attitude and for funding to be channelled to ensure that equal rights are automatically available to all disabled people.

Ironically, it would probably be cheaper, in the long run, if a concerted effort were made to produce environmental adaptations and ensure equal rights implementation, instead of relying on the rather piecemeal funding which is currently available.

Having said all this, if you really feel the need for some specific equipment or group activity, using charitable funding is one way of possibly gaining access to it.

If you cannot get funding from the local authority the next step is to contact appropriate charities who may be able to offer grants. (Your local library will have a list of grant-making trusts.) Groups can make applications to national appeals such as 'Children in Need' run by the BBC, and local private businesses can sometimes be persuaded to make donations, especially to help group efforts.

If all else fails you might wish to consider a fund raising effort organised by yourself or by local people. Sponsored events are the most popular, such as sponsored runs, swims, bike rides, dances (anything). Other ways to raise funds privately include market stalls, raffles, stalls at Christmas or summer fêtes, collecting boxes in pubs or shops. It should be remembered that these events often involve a lot of effort for very little financial reward, but they may tip the balance to enable you to purchase much needed equipment or services. I recently came across a simple and easy to organise method of raising money which might be of interest. If you ask 10 people to find 10 people each who would be willing to donate £10 you will raise £1000. To make this effective it is a good idea to produce an information sheet (with a photo on it if possible) so that the collectors can show this to people they are requesting donations from.

To give fund raising legitimacy it is preferable for you to be collecting money under a registered charity number. There are some organisations who will act as an 'umbrella' for individuals wishing to raise money to meet their children's special needs. Alternatively, you can get together with other parents or individually set up a charity. Setting up a charity is not easy and you would be advised to seek an easier option than setting up an individual charity for one child. Group efforts are often more successful than lone activity.

When you are raising money you need to be fairly careful how you phrase information about what the money is being raised for. If you specify a very narrow option for spending the money and then find that the facility you are raising money for is no longer available you may be legally barred from using the money to serve other needs your child may have. On the other hand, it is imperative that money is spent on activities or items which would be considered charitable. When raising money for Danny I usually either specify a range of options for which the money will be used or make a general statement that the money raised will be used to benefit his development.

## Community care

Community care is a term which was coined in the 1950s to describe the need to move away from the tendency to keep people with disabilities in institutions and to provide opportunities for integration within the community. In the early days the emphasis was on replacing large institutions housing children. More recently, community care has become associated with the replacement of long-stay hospitals for people with mental health problems, learning difficulties, physical disabilities or elderly people.

It is rare these days for a child born with disabilities to be removed into an institution. Instead, the child is more likely to live with her natural family. Community care is receiving a great deal of publicity at the moment as many long-stay hospitals are being closed down and people who have been living in them are being moved into the community.

There has been a great deal of research commissioned by successive governments to tackle the issues but very little money has been made available to facilitate the desired move towards integration into the community. Resources which go into community care projects are always aimed at taking people out of institutions and supporting them in the community.

In 1976, joint finance was made available to health and local authorities so that they could jointly plan and pay for the development of community care services to be run by the local authorities. In 1983 the Health and Social Services and Social Securities (Adjudications) Act introduced the care in the community initiative aimed at moving people out of long-stay hospitals and returning them to the community. In 1985 the House of Commons Social Services Committee recommended that closure of long-stay hospitals should be slowed down because the alternative services could not be demonstrated to be adequate.

Various reports have been commissioned since 1985 and the recommendations are broadly similar:

- That people with disabilities should be able to make a positive choice about their living situation;
- That local authorities should provide the necessary support to enable individuals to live in the community with dignity (for example, having their own key to their own room, access to their own money from which they pay rent etc.; assistance with representation to statutory authorities to ensure that complaints are fairly heard).

In April 1988, the House of Commons Committee of Public Accounts concluded that local authorities had been reluctant to take up joint finance, that the DHSS was failing to exercise proper financial control over joint finance schemes, that arrangements for monitoring residential homes were unsatisfactory and that the implementation of community care projects was likely to be adversely affected by a shortage of nursing and therapy professionals.

The Government's current Key Objectives for community care are as follows:

- To promote the development of domiciliary, day and respite services to enable people to live in their own homes wherever feasible and sensible;
- To ensure that service providers make practical support for carers a high priority;
- To make proper assessment of need and good case management the cornerstone of high quality care;
- To promote the development of a flourishing independent sector alongside good quality public services;
- To clarify the responsibilities of agencies and so make it easier to hold them to account for their performance;
- To secure better value for taxpayers' money by introducing a new funding structure for social care.

In order to achieve these objectives the Government proposes to make a number of changes in the way in which social care is delivered and funded:

- Local authorities are to become responsible, in collaboration with health and other interested services, for assessing need and providing care arrangements within available resources;
- Local authorities are expected to produce and publish clear plans for the development of community care services;
- Local authorities will be expected to make maximum use of the independent sector;
- Local authorities are to become responsible for the financial support of people in private and voluntary homes, over and above any general social security entitlements;
- Applicants with few or no resources of their own will be eligible for the same levels of Income Support and Housing Benefit, irrespective of whether they are living in their own homes or in independent residential or nursing homes;
- Inspection and registration units are to be set up within local authorities to check on standards in all residential care homes;
- There will be a new specific grant to promote the development of social care for seriously mentally ill people.

## Resources for community care

People entering residential or nursing homes who need financial support will be able to claim Income Support and Housing Benefit, as if they were in their own homes. Local authorities will pay the full cost and reclaim it from residents' social security payments.

Local authorities will receive the resources previously allocated by social security to residents in private and voluntary homes. Additional resources will be distributed through the Revenue Support Grant.

Health Authorities will continue to fund mainstream community care activities from their own resources.

For children with disabilities community care starts (and usually stays) in the home. The carer is often the parent with little or no support automatically on offer and a lack of information about the rights of the family or where extra help can be obtained.

The early needs of your child in the community are likely to be identified by the paediatric consultant or health visitor. The expertise of these professionals may be geared towards physical and medical care and treatment rather than the social needs of the child. There are a number of professionals and voluntary agencies to which the carer of a young child who has disabilities can turn for help, advice and support. My own research suggests, however, that many carers never even discover the existence of such voluntary agencies, and often do not get any contact from professionals in the community until their child is older or unless a family crisis occurs.

You may be offered access to a specialist, a peripatetic teacher, a social worker, a play group geared up to meet your child's needs, respite care (where you feel that your child is satisfactorily looked after while you get a rest), counselling or voluntary agencies in your area. If you are not offered any of these resources, *you should feel able to ask for them.* Your consultant can often refer you for some of the services. The local branch of Scope might be able to put you in contact with voluntary agencies in your area. The local town hall should have a register of voluntary agencies, and your nearest Citizens' Advice Bureau can also help.

## Support in the home

There are a number of voluntary and statutory services available to provide various kinds of support in the home but, like all services, they are often in short supply and with long waiting lists. The kind of help you can get under statutory obligation is listed in Chapter 9.

Each area will have its own emphasis and availability of various forms of help. You should be able to get advice from the health visitor or Social Services about statutory (and sometimes voluntary) services available in your area. Alternatively you can contact the local branch of Scope. The following are examples of the kind of help which might be available:

**Crossroads**   Crossroads is a national network which provides care attendants for set periods to go into the home on a regular basis to take the place of full-time carers of disabled relatives and friends while the carer gets a break. The provision of a Crossroads care attendant allows the carer to have a few hours break a week, just enough to free her for a short while, to add extra help in a crisis, or as an insurance against breakdown.

Initially your needs would be assessed by a management worker from the local office and, once it has been established that the service meets your need, you go on a waiting list until a care attendant's time becomes available. Whenever possible Crossroads try to ensure that the family has the continuity of one care attendant whom they get to know and who can develop an understanding of the needs and interests of the person being cared for.

**Community Service Volunteers (CSV)**   This is a national volunteering scheme which offers work experience opportunities to young people for a set period of time. Volunteers are recruited in a number of different ways under different schemes run by CSV. Under some schemes unemployed or socially disadvantaged young people might use CSV as an opportunity to get work experience on a part-time basis while they also explore other opportunities such as part-time training courses etc. These volunteers might go into schools, day centres, play groups or residential centres to support the activities going on there.

The Independent Living Project (organised by CSV) is a full-time volunteering scheme whereby the young person contracts to work full-time for a specified number of months on an individual project. These schemes cost the authority or project a certain amount of money (approximately £7000 per annum by 1991 prices) as the volunteer must have accommodation provided, food paid for and a specified amount of spending money per week as well as supervision from Social Services (or another professional as appropriate). In return for this they will give 35–40 hours per week to whatever project they are allocated to. An example of the Independent Living Project is living in the home of an adult with disabilities to facilitate his independence in the home so that he can live in the community rather than in assisted, residential care. If the adult needs assistance 24 hours a day, it can take up to three volunteers to service one person. More recently there has been an interest (in some areas) in expanding the Independent Living Project arrangements where a volunteer goes and lives with a family where there is a child who has disabilities. The main purpose of placing a volunteer in the home of a child who has disabilities is to increase the child's opportunity of getting stimulation and all possible help in her development. CSV volunteers can also be placed in schools to help out generally or to facilitate the pupils who have special needs.

**Getting help**   If you are interested in the possibility of getting help through CSV there are a number of points which you should consider first:

- Community service volunteering is a two-way process. The project gets help for a reasonable financial outlay but there is a need to be considerate of the volunteers' need to gain in terms of work experience and personal development. Are you able to support the volunteer at the same time as receiving support yourself?
- CSV projects need to be funded. In some cases the local authority will provide funding, otherwise you would be reliant on fund raising or your own resources. Where the finance will come from needs careful consideration.
- The local Social Services Department or another appropriate agency must be willing to support the project at least in offering supervision for the volunteer. This would probably involve a social worker (or similarly qualified professional) in about one hour per fortnight meeting with the volunteer and generally monitoring the project.

## Private agencies

If you have the resources there are a number of private agencies which operate throughout the country who offer qualified nurses to come and take over your caring role for regular or occasional periods depending on your need.

## Voluntary agencies and what they offer

There are a huge number of voluntary agencies which have been set up to provide support for children with disabilities (see the list of useful addresses and contacts on pages 219–231). Some are national organisations and others are locally based. You should be able to find out about your local voluntary agencies from Citizens' Advice Bureaux, the Town Hall, the local library, the local branch of Scope or the local church.

Voluntary agencies attempt to offer direct support (such as relief for carers, holidays for children who have disabilities, play schemes, financial assistance), or advice on financial assistance and family support networks.

## Charities

There are numerous charities which give financial aid to individual children in need. Many other charities prefer to give money to groups set up to help children in need. There are several publications which detail such charities and what they might be willing to assist with (see the list of useful addresses and contacts on pages 219–231).

# Institutionalised care

In 1970, it was estimated that there were 146,500 children under the age of 16 who were 'deprived of a normal family life'. Of these approximately 19,000 were children with disabilities. The number of children in institutionalised care number between 80,000 and 90,000. These children live in establishments where they are cared for by paid staff in an environment which is organised very differently from that of an ordinary home or foster home. A disproportionate number of children with disabilities reside in such care situations.

Studies have shown that the organisation of mental handicap hospitals and some of the long-stay units for other types of disability compares very unfavourably with that of homes for non-disabled children. Residential care is very far removed from any notion of integration between non-disabled and disabled people. The extreme of segregation tends to occur in residential care. Children with disabilities are very often brought up in institutions which are specially set aside for them rather than in ordinary children's homes. A child's world is largely shaped by the adults who care for him. In institutional-ised care this is likely to be a constant stream of ever changing, underpaid staff who cannot afford the time or the emotional drain of forming a bond with the individual child whom they will inevitably leave when they move on to alternative employment.

It has been found that child care practices differ according to the size of institutions rather than the severity of a child's disability – i.e. the larger the institution the less personalised the care.

With the introduction of community care there is a greater drive than ever before to enable people, wherever possible, to live in the community. Many older people who have CP have lived in institutionalised care (some in long-stay hospitals for the mentally subnormal) all of their lives. A huge proportion of these people could have been living in their own homes, or in appropriately supported shared homes.

Scope runs a number of residential homes, originally set up as an alternative to the conventional institutions. However, the emphasis in these homes has changed enormously in recent years and residents are now encouraged to have much greater access to the wider community.

The development of specialist Housing Associations, provid-ing specially adapted housing for people with disabilities, offers one solution but there are not nearly enough of such dwellings to meet the demand.

# 7

# Education

'Hello. I am a disabled boy. I wish to be understood and may I tell you my feelings. We may be disabled but we have our abilities too. I always believe the value of life is not measured by the length of life but by what one can achieve during life.

'A good friend of mine once said "Life is like a comet, it will lighten up and brighten the whole world, even though it may sparkle and disappear in a second".

'I wish people would give us the opportunity to reach our potential. I, too, sincerely hope all the disabled could understand the meaning of those words and try their best to contribute to their society.'

Wong Chi Hang, aged 15

Education is the cornerstone of our future lives. It is the key which opens the door to all future possibilities.

Everything we are able to do as adults is the result of what we learnt as children. This includes the value we put upon ourselves as human beings as well as our social standing and ability to be financially and domestically independent and to fulfil our ambitions.

The kind of education we receive can empower or disempower depending on where we are taught, what we are taught, by whom we are taught and with what end in view.

It is important to consider what needs a child will have as an adult, when he is being entered into the education system. This is especially so if the child has a disability. If you are aiming only to give your child social and domestic independence and not giving consideration to academic achievement then his chances of obtaining gainful and rewarding employment are limited. If you consider only the child's academic opportunities then chances of independent living might be limited.

# Pre-school learning

Pre-school learning opportunities are particularly helpful to children who have disabilities, and local authorities have a statutory obligation to consider the special educational needs of children with disabilities who are under the age of 5.

Whatever the extent of your child's disability, he will be helped by a little extra preparation before entering full-time education. There are a number of statutory options which might be available in your area. Alternatively, you can find out about pre-school learning and spend some time preparing your child yourself. Another option is to get together with other parents who have pre-school children and gather mutual support in offering your children pre-school opportunities.

## Pre-school nurseries

There is a fairly short supply of pre-school nursery places available in this country. Recent estimates are that places are available for only 2 per cent of the pre-school population. Availability of places varies from area to area. Your Local Education Authority should be able to advise you about which institutions to approach. Nurseries are sometimes attached to primary schools and it is worth considering entering your child in a nursery at a school he is likely to attend long term if at all possible. Some nurseries operate separately from local schools. Many of these are funded by the local authority although there has been a recent increase in the number of privately run nurseries.

If your child is recognised as having special educational needs at an early age you may be entitled to high priority for a nursery placement. Your local Social Services or Education Department will be able to advise you about this.

## Preparing at home

Peripatetic teachers are available in some areas but they are unfortunately in short supply. Ask your education department if they can offer you this facility. The local educational psychologist may also be able to offer advice on this. Peripatetic teachers who are trained in special education can visit on a regular basis and offer advice on how best to prepare your child for full-time education. Some teachers use specific training programmes, such as Portage, for children with disabilities. Some teachers may specialise in hearing or visual impairment, or both.

## The Portage early education programme

Portage is a system for assessing the needs of young people who have developmental delay and then teaching them the skills they need to acquire. It is a home-centred system which involves regular home visits from a member of the multidisciplinary team running the service. The home visit provides an opportunity for parents to seek guidance, discuss needs and set learning targets for their child. The parent is recognised as the key figure in a child's development and the Portage system is designed to help parents to focus on their child's abilities and learning needs and carry out tasks which will aid his progress.

A number of Local Education Authorities have either already adopted the Portage system or are considering doing so. Given that there is currently very little cohesive and structured advice available to parents who wish to help their children to develop in their early years this can only be a good thing. However, it would be unfortunate if Local Education Authorities were to feel that they had fully discharged their duty in relation to pre-school children who have special needs by adopting Portage. Portage is a system which should be available to parents and children but not to the exclusion of other early educational opportunities. As the system is carried out in the home between parent and child, there is no facility for interaction with other children. Also, it was originally designed for children with quite specific learning difficulties and the system is now being generalised.

More information about Portage can be found through the useful addresses and contacts list, given on page 219.

## Mother and toddler groups

Find out if there is a local mother and toddler group your child can attend with you. This will give him an early chance to interact with non-disabled children and to learn from group play activities.

# Conductive education

This is a pre-school learning system especially designed for children with motor impairment and aims to give them the opportunity to enter normal school with reduced disability.

## The background to conductive education

The main aim of conductive education is to produce *orthofunction* (ability to satisfy biological and social demands) in children with motor disorders so that they can take up places in Hungarian general or special schools. However, it is a system which is receiving unprecedented publicity with a huge lobby of parents pushing for its swift introduction in Britain. The system was devised in Hungary during the 1950s by Andres Peto (a physician who specialised in institutions of rehabilitation). Conductive education was devised in a very different culture where the demands of the education system and the economic climate vary greatly from Britain. The importance of being able to walk is emphasised because, under the Hungarian education system, children who are unable to walk cannot attend either a general or a special school. For these children teaching tends to be home-based which is unsatisfactory and costly. Conductive education is not a long-term alternative to meet the educational needs of children otherwise unable to manage in the general school system. It specifically aims to remediate motor and other learning difficulties experienced by certain groups of children with the aim of discharging them into the general school system.

Peto set up a National Institute for Kinesitherapy in 1950. By 1963 the institute had become the 'Institute for Training of Educators of the Locomotor Handicapped and the Educational Home for the Locomotor Handicapped'. It was here that he began training conductors in the system which is used today.

After Peto's death in 1967, Dr Maria Hari took over as Director of the Institute, a position she still holds today. A new Institute has now been established in Budapest since 1985 and is called 'The Andres Peto Institute for Motor Disorders'. Since 1963, the Peto Institute has provided a statutory service for all school children in Hungary who have disorders for which conductive education is felt to be an appropriate remedial method.

There has been wide criticism of the method – mainly due to lack of scientific data, research papers or general written work from Hungary to enable the system to be evaluated. However, it is generally acknowledged as being successful in creating 'orthofunction' in pupils who attend.

Scope began to take a serious interest in the work of the Peto Institute in the late 1960s and early 1970s, and since the 1960s some British children have been taken to Hungary for assessment and training. Ester Cotton (a physiotherapist who was working for Scope) provided the initial force in developing conductive education in this country. Inspired by the work at the Peto Institute she produced a system of pre-school motor training designed to enable young children to acquire 'basic motor patterns' essential for full physical function. Her system is not conductive education but uses techniques found within conductive education under the influence of a conductive philosophy.

In 1992 Scope reached an agreement with the Peto Institute in Hungary. Initial assessments for British children are now available at the Peto Andres Centre for Conductive Education located at the Fitzroy Square assessment centre run by Scope in London. Hungarian conductors work at the centre as well as British ones. If the conductors believe that conductive education will be of benefit to a child they have the opportunity to be referred to one of a number of options. These may include follow up courses at Fitzroy Square, contact with a school for parents or a visit to Hungary for an intensive course.

Local schools for parents are being set up by Scope to act as centres where parents of young children can learn about the principles of conductive education, explore other options and learn ways of helping their children at home.

For more information about the Peto Andres Centre you can ring the Cerebral Palsy helpline (see useful addresses page 219).

There are a number of independent centres springing up around the country who aim to offer techniques inspired by conductive education. Some of these centres are employing Peto trained conductors. There are also some conductors working independently. The Foundation for Conductive Education in Birmingham may be able to give further information on local activity around the country.

The Hornsey Centre, and independent school at Haringay, London, which was set up to provide pre-school learning opportunities for children with cerebral palsy has tailored the emphasis of its work over the last 3–4 years and is now carrying out training programmes designed to replicate the work of the Peto institute. The Hornsey Centre is advised by a trained conductor from Hungary and by Ester Cotton.

In recent years there has been an upsurge in the number of Hungarian trained conductors entering this country and seeking to offer their services both privately and to various institutions and schools.

In 1984 The Birmingham Institute for Conductive Education was formed. The Birmingham Institute aims to bring conductive education into Britain in a systematised way which will enable, as near as possible, a true replication of the work of the Peto Institute in this country. In 1987 ten trainee conductors, all of them holding British teaching qualifications, were recruited. At the same time ten children, all of whom have cerebral palsy, were selected with the help of two Hungarian conductors to be the first intake into the Birmingham Institute. The children and trainee conductors spend part of their time working in this country under the direction of Hungarian conductors and part of their time working in Hungary. Further children continue to be assessed and trainee conductors recruited as the work of the Birmingham Institute expands. A second institute is being developed in Scotland with support from the Birmingham Institute and the Peto Institute.

It will be a long time before conductive education is widely available in this country. The arrangement which Scope has made with the Peto Institute at least enables children to have initial assessments in this country but a full conductive programme may still require visits to Hungary of varying lengths in the near future. To enable children to have the opportunity to benefit from visits to Hungary, the British Government has contributed £5m towards the establishing of an international school for conductive education to be developed in Hungary. In addition to this, local authorities have been given legislative powers to provide funding for individual children to visit centres abroad which may help their educational progress.

## How does conductive education work?

Andres Peto considered motor disorder as a learning difficulty to be overcome rather than a condition which requires treatment or accommodation. He set out to establish motor function in young children which would diminish or eradicate physical handicap which might otherwise persist into adult life. It is also intended that overcoming motor disorder through an integrated learning programme will facilitate the child in all aspects of development (e.g. intellectual function and personality development). Conductive education has been found to be helpful to children and adults with a number of 'conditions' which involve motor dysfunction. These include cerebral palsy, spina bifida, stroke and Parkinson's disease.

It is the educational emphasis of the system which sets it apart from other methods which have been devised to help children who have cerebral palsy in their development. The context is a learning one in which the child uses her own efforts to overcome her problems under the guidance of a trained conductor. The will and determination of the pupil play a central role in the success of the system and the training is designed to take place within the wider context of a general education system for all.

Another important aspect of conductive education is that almost all of the learning takes place in groups. Children are matched in groups and learn together. Each child's achievements are noted and appreciated by the group as a whole. In addition to the incentive of group support, development is aided by the example set by the achievements of peers.

Motivation is important and devices are employed to aid the development of motivation through song, rhyme, the use of toys etc. as well as highlighting the achievements of children who have done well and giving appreciation to other children and conductors.

Children who attend the Peto Institute go through an intensive day during which every activity of daily life is an opportunity for education. Those who are resident at the Institute begin their day by being woken by a conductor who will help them with dressing and toilet before breakfast. Independence is the ultimate goal of every task. Where children require assistance from a conductor this is kept to a minimum and the children may also help each other in basic tasks such as dressing. Slatted benches are used for most activities (such as dressing, washing and eating) as the slats in the bench maximise self-help, enabling the children to steady themselves and retain balance. At about 9 am children will begin the daily routine of 'lessons' generally known as 'task series'. Task series teach the performance of tasks learned spontaneously by healthy children. They are neither simple exercises nor defined anatomical movements but intentional activities in a biological sense. These might include sitting, grasping and other hand control activities and ultimately standing and walking. The children learn in a group and demonstrate their intention verbally. For example, the child may say 'I stretch my right hand back' while the conductor aids the child to undertake the task. The next part of the task might be 'I stretch it down again', and so on, culminating in 'I clap my hands'. Day by day the level of achievement required by the schedule rises. Task series represent the path which is seen to lead to orthofunction. They are goal directed and carefully constructed to meet the function needs of the specific group of individuals undertaking them. Task series learning is interspersed with 'conditioning' (e.g. toilet training, washing, eating etc.) The process continues up until lights out at 9 pm.

A typical day at the Birmingham Institute, where children attend on a daily basis rather than boarding, will begin at 8.30 am with changing and potty training. A lying-down programme might follow with further potty training then refreshments after this. During the day there will be various programmes aimed at walking, sitting, speech and preparation for school with toilet, washing and eating interspersed at regular intervals throughout until the end of the day at 5 pm.

## Criticisms of the system: positive and negative aspects

A number of Scope schools and other institutions have taken some elements of the conductive system into the daily teaching programmes they practise but the level of intensity and exact similarity to the method as it is carried out in Hungary varies widely. There is a four year training required before a conductor is fully qualified and many of those programmes being taught which have been inspired by the Peto Institute are not being administered by trained conductors. Where trained conductors are employed there may not be the facilities or desire for the intensity of programme which exists in Hungary or at the Birmingham Institute. It is therefore very difficult to judge the effectiveness of programmes inspired by conductive education since there appear to be differences in the approaches of the different institutions.

I do not wish to discredit institutions or individual conductors who are offering programmes based on conductive education rather than fully implementing it in practice. Many children have benefited from working in this way. Advice from someone with a conductive orientation can have a positive influence on the parental handling – for example, ensuring that the child's day incorporates training such as potty training, self-help at meal times, sitting and standing practice, symmetry in all activities and repetition sufficient to enable real learning to take place.

There have been many criticisms of conductive education made by therapists who operate from different traditions. These include the following:

- The system is exclusive, only taking children who have demonstrated certain intellectual and physical abilities prior to training. The success rate is only so high because of the 'weeding out' of more severely disabled children in the early stages.
- The high demands of the training are too great for small children to cope with.
- Reliance on one professional to facilitate all aspects of a child's development can only lead to a less skilled professional in individual areas of development such as speech.

There may be some truth in all of these criticisms. There may also be some professional jealousy involved where 'experts' in other traditions feel that their systems and beliefs are threatened by conductive education.

At the end of the day it is up to the child and the parent (as advocate of the child) to follow up the systems of their choice and draw their own conclusions. The following quote is from Graham Chambers, whose little boy Lawrence graduated from the Birmingham Institute in June 1989 and went on to attend the local infants school.

'The best prognosis we had had before he started the Institute was that within about 12 months he would be walking. Within three months not only was he walking but he was walking considerable distances ... correcting his balance, he was able to turn and move off in a different direction. From Lawrence's point of view this released the frustration that he felt ... being unable to compete with his brothers and sisters ... That in itself has helped us as a family. ...'

I have met adults with cerebral palsy who heavily criticise conductive education for detracting from the real issues of the need for better access in society and improved provision of aids and adaptations. They also criticise the régime as cruel and yet another attempt to force the person with disabilities to fit into society rather than society adapting. This is a long standing dilemma and conflict which will continue to surround the issue of provision for people with disabilities. There is no easy solution and I do not intend to propose one in this publication. I would only suggest that every person who has disabilities deserves the right of access to whatever form of support may be available and desired by that person to facilitate their equal and full participation in the community.

## Entering your child into the general education system

### The law and education for children with disabilities

Section 36 of the 1944 Education Act requires parents to ensure that their children 'receive education suited to their age, ability and aptitude, either by regular attendance at school or otherwise'. Section 8 of the same Act places a duty on local authorities 'that there shall be available sufficient (primary and secondary) schools to provide full time education for junior and senior pupils.'

Parents and local authorities have a duty to ensure that appropriate education is made available to children from the age of 5 to the age of 16. There are many provisions in the 1944 and subsequent Education Acts which enable parents to exercise choice regarding the education of their children. However, if your child has a disability you may find that the process of entering your child into the education system is fraught with complexity. One of the biggest debates in the area of disability at the present time is around the options of segregated versus integrated education for children with disabilities – i.e. whether to send your child to a special school or to a mainstream school.

The educational needs of children with disabilities (in education the most commonly used phrase is 'children with special educational needs') was not enshrined in legislation until the 1944 Education Act. This Act laid down that all pupils should be afforded 'opportunities for education offering such variety of instruction and training as may be desirable in view of their different ages, abilities and aptitudes, and of the different periods for which they might be expected to remain at school'. Eleven categories of handicap were defined in the Act: blind, partially sighted, deaf, partially deaf, delicate, diabetic, educationally subnormal, epileptic, maladjusted, physically handicapped and those with speech defects. The 1944 Act was interpreted by the Ministry of Education as promoting the education of children with special needs in special schools. The emphasis changed in 1978 when the Warnock Committee reported on the education of handicapped children and young persons. The Warnock Report recommended that special provision should be additional or supplementary to general education rather than a separate or alternative provision. The 1981 Education Act came about partly in response to the Warnock Report and was meant to emphasise the integration of children with special educational needs into mainstream educational institutions. However, many supporters of integration maintain that the Act fell short in that there are too many loopholes which enable local authorities to avoid integration.

Section 36 of the 1944 Education Act was amended to include a duty of parents to cause their child to receive education suitable to 'any special educational needs he may have'. The 1981 Act also placed a duty on local authorities for identification, assessment and provision for children 'whose special educational needs call for the authority to determine the special educational provision'. A duty was laid on Health Authorities to bring any likely special educational needs of children under 5 to the attention of the appropriate education authority.

According to the legal definitions, a child has a learning difficulty if he or she has:

- 'Significantly greater difficulty in learning than the majority of children of his age';
- 'Has a disability which either prevents or hinders him from making use of educational facilities of a kind generally provided in schools, within the area of the local authority concerned, for children of his age'; or
- 'Is aged under 5 and is likely to fall into one of these categories when over 5, or is likely to unless special educational provision is made.'

**Special educational provision** Special educational provision for children under 2 means *any* educational provision, and for children aged 2 and over it means 'educational provision which is additional to or otherwise different from the education provision made generally for children of his age in schools maintained by the local authority concerned'.

A child has special educational needs if he or she has a learning difficulty which calls for a special educational provision to be made.

The most significant change which the 1981 Act made in meeting the needs of children with disabilities was to promote the education of children with special needs in ordinary schools alongside children without special needs. This duty applies to *all* children whatever their particular disability and however severe it may be. However, three conditions were included which considerably water down the effectiveness of this piece of legislation as described below.

Children with special educational needs are to be educated in ordinary schools, provided that account has been taken of parents' views, and education in an ordinary school is compatible with:

- The child receiving the special educational provision which he or she requires;
- The provision of 'efficient education' for children with whom he or she will be educated;
- The efficient use of resources.

Finally, the 1981 Act states that the involvement of the child's parents is essential. Assessment should be seen as a partnership between teachers, other professionals and parents. This adds to the overriding principle outlined in the 1944 Act that 'so far as is compatible with the provision of efficient instruction and training and the avoidance of unreasonable public expenditure, pupils are to be educated in accordance with the wishes of their parents.'

## The 1993 Education Act and the 1994 Code of Practice

The 1993 Education Act follows the 1981 Act and is a substantial piece of legislation. The Code of Practice explains how the part of the Act which relates to special educational needs ought to be implemented. From September 1995, all schools should be following the Code of Practice. They should also have published their *Special Educational Needs Policy* so you should be able to request one.

These are some of the key points in the Act and the Code of Practice:

● Time scales for assessments have been introduced to speed up the statementing process.
● A new style of tribunal will have more powers to enforce decisions.
● The importance of consulting parents and taking children's views seriously is emphasised.
● Early assessments are recommended i.e. assessments for 2–5 year olds which will help get resources for a child before she is in school.
● Where 'appropriate' and where parents wish it, children with special needs should be educated in mainstream schools.

Unfortunately, for many parents who want local mainstream schools for their children, the Code of Practice may not go far enough as parents still have to prove that their child's place in the school will be a good use of resources, will not affect other children's education and that their child's needs can be met in school. If parents need help and support from organisations campaigning for inclusive education see useful addresses and contacts on page 219.

## The law in practice

**Statementing**   There are formal procedures for assessing a child's special educational needs. Once the assessment procedure has been carried out, and if your child is deemed to have special educational needs, a statement of these needs will be produced. The statement is a legal document and the local authority is required to make whatever provision is deemed necessary in the statement. The procedure is often known as 'statementing'.

Anyone can request an assessment who has direct involvement with the child's developmental needs (and this includes parents). The procedure is started with a formal letter to the Education Officer requesting that they assess the needs of your child. You are not obliged to give reasons for the request but it is normal practice and common sense to do so. Reasons might include a few words about the nature of the child's disability and the intentions of the parents, where known, regarding their child's education. If the Education Authority refuses to make an assessment you can consider making a formal complaint to the Secretary of State for Education.

Once the authority has decided that an assessment should take place they must send the parents a formal notice which informs them of the intention to assess, the procedures which are to be followed, the name of an officer they may go to for further information and their rights to make representations which must be within a period of 29 days from the date the notice is served.

From here on the amount of actual involvement a parent is invited to have in the procedure will differ from one local authority to another. You should ensure that you are satisfied with the reasons for assessment and ask to see any written documents which are produced regarding your child's needs as well as which professionals the local authority intend to consult. If case conferences are to be held you should ask when these are likely to take place and request permission to attend.

It is usual for the local educational psychologist to prepare the final statement but a broad range of views should be sought from professionals involved with your child as well as the parents. The professionals consulted are likely to include any or all of the following: physiotherapist, occupational therapist, any teaching staff who have been involved with your child, speech and language therapist, consultant or GP, Social Services representatives. The parent may request that any relevant person is consulted. For example, you may wish to involve private therapists (if you have been seeing one) or play leaders (if your child has been attending a play group) etc. If you feel that you are not in agreement with a professional who is seeing your child on a regular basis you should seek independent advice as quickly as possible (see the useful addresses and contacts section on page 219 for further information).

Ideally, a statement should protect your child by ensuring that he receives the provision necessary to enable him to get the best out of the education system. However, the statement is something of a double edged sword in that parents of children with statements are excluded from the right to express a preference for a particular school as laid down in the 1980

Education Act. Until your child has a statement you can exercise your right to express a preference for a particular 'ordinary' school and appeal to a local appeal committee if you are refused a place. However, the statement removes this right.

On the one hand you may desire a statement of your child's needs. If your child's disability is severe you will need to have a statement in order to gain access to services. On the other hand, if the provision determined by the statement is not in accord with your wishes you are put in a very difficult position.

It is advisable to be clear on your preferences regarding your child's education before the statementing procedure begins and it will greatly assist your case if you have professionals or teachers whose views accord with your own also providing reports.

There have been a number of newspaper articles in recent years where local authorities have been accused of abusing the statementing procedure by writing statements which are tailored to the availability of certain provisions rather than the educational needs of the child. For example, if you live in an area where there is a high density of special schools it might be tempting for the local authority to provide a statement recommending your child should attend a special school even if you believe it is not in your child's interests. If you want your child to attend a mainstream school it is important that you gather arguments which are based on the law. You need to demonstrate that the attendance of your child at the school of your choice will best enable her to receive the special educational provision she needs, will not detract from the efficient education of the children with whom she will be educated and will represent an efficient use of resources. In an area where resources for children with special educational needs are concentrated in special schools, this latter point may be difficult to press. In areas where the roll in special schools is declining there may be even more incentive on the part of the local authority to pressure parents into sending their children to special schools.

As well as naming the institution in which your child should receive education, the statement will lay down specific therapy, training aids, any extra teaching or care, support and equipment which should be provided by the local authority. The Advisory Centre for Education (ACE – see the list of useful addresses and contacts on page 219) can offer advice and support to parents whose children are going through the statementing procedure. They also produce a handbook, *The ACE Special Education Handbook: The Law on Children and Special Needs*. This can be obtained from ACE.

## Making a choice about your child's education

If your child is only mildly affected it is unlikely that he will require a statement and you will probably choose to send him to a local mainstream school in the normal way. However, the majority of children with cerebral palsy are likely to have some special educational needs and it is important that you are clear about your choice of education for your child as early as possible so that appropriate arrangements can be made for his needs to be met successfully.

The main choices are currently between special schools, mainstream schools and special units in mainstream schools.

## The special school system

It is important that the place of special schooling is seen in its historical context. Special schools were set up, mainly in the 1970s, in response to new legislation which gave all disabled children the right to receive education for the first time in history. Previously, disabled children had either managed to cope, without extra support, in the ordinary schools, or had been sent away to 'caring' institutions or had been kept at home by families who did their best for their children in whatever way they could. Initially then, the opportunity to go off to school, albeit a special one, seemed like a great step forward. However, we are now left with a legacy from these schools which is proving to be the great educational dilemma for disabled children in the 1990s and beyond. The distinction between education and therapy must be understood and recognised. The special school system tends to mesh these two needs together, often prioritising therapy over education to the detriment of academic outcome.

Some special schools are boarding schools and, in many cases, the special school most appropriate for your child will be outside the local area. The distances children have to travel and the lack of contact with their peers in the local community which travelling to a special school produces are two of the many arguments which are levelled against special school provision. Other arguments include the following:

- Special school education is essentially segregated education. The child is kept away from her local community and educated amongst other children who have special educational needs. Every child who has a disability is a unique individual so the grouping together of children with disabilities does not necessarily ensure that your child will be receiving an education which is better suited to her needs than that which is available at a local mainstream school.
- The environment of the special school is very separate from that of the general community. Sooner or later your child will be expected to take a full part in her local community. A child who has been kept in a segregated community until the age of 19 is ill equipped to deal with the outside world.
- Special schools may tend to underestimate a child's abilities and it is possible that education will be tailored more towards domestic and social skills than towards academic achievement.

Arguments in favour of special schooling usually go along the following lines:

- Resources being concentrated in one place enable a child to have more ready access to other services. For example, most special schools will have physiotherapy departments and regular input from other relevant health professionals. (I have also, however, heard many parents of children who attend special schools complain bitterly that they feel their children do not receive sufficient time and attention from the School Health Service and that their own involvement in their child's health care is diminished by the concentration of therapeutic activities within the school.)
- Special schools are meant to be readily equipped with aids and adaptations as well as specialised teaching equipment and specially trained teachers.

## Mainstream school

The successful enjoyment your child will have of education at mainstream schools will depend on a number of factors. The extent of your child's disability and the amount of 'extra' help he is likely to need will be of prime concern to the school. If your child's disability is mild with little or no extra help needed the main concern is likely to be the attitudes of non-disabled peers and teachers towards him. Because disability is still so hidden in our society it is an unfortunate fact that negative images pervade in society. Cruel remarks and bullying from other children can become a common occurrence. However, children do not behave in this way spontaneously. They learn such behaviour from adults and images around them in society. A positive attitude from teachers (and particularly head teachers) can do much to overcome this. So can contact with and support from other parents. At the end of the day people with disabilities will not avoid the pain of negative attitudes from others by being hidden away. It is only by full and continued participation in society, coupled with positive legislation, that attitudes can be made to change.

If your child's disability is severe it will probably be necessary for you to obtain a statement of his needs so that proper provision can be made within the mainstream setting. It is theoretically possible for the local authority to provide your child with a helper in school to enable him in having both his physical needs met and aiding him in carrying out lessons. However, limited financial resources are very stretched for this kind of help and, if your child is likely to need this kind of help full-time, the local authority may try and argue that your child should be catered for in a special school.

There are various theories on the best way to enable integration. My own position is that integration begins at birth and should perhaps be renamed 'participation'. In recent years a growing movement, largely led by disabled adults and parents of disabled children, has coined the term 'inclusive education' arguing that what is required is for the child to be included fully in their communities and that the term 'integration' does not represent this need. If children with disabilities are invited and encouraged to take a full place in society from the start of their lives there is no reason to suppose that they will not be able to take their place beside non-disabled peers in all walks of life and all activities.

Seamus Hegarty in his book *Special Needs in Ordinary Schools* makes the point the term 'integration' is potentially misleading and may divert from the real task to be done.

'What pupils who have difficulties need is *education*, not

integration. Placing them in an ordinary school is not an end in itself but a means toward the end of securing them an appropriate education.'

The impression is created that it is the pupil who must adapt to the school system rather than the school making appropriate changes to accommodate the needs of the pupil. Success tends to be measured against how well children with special needs are absorbed into mainstream rather than how mainstream has adapted to accommodate them.

In order for a mainstream school to be able to offer full educational opportunities to children who have special educational needs it is essential that staff are prepared and trained to be enablers for these pupils. If you are considering a mainstream school you should talk to the head about the attitude of the school towards children with disabilities and find out if there are any teachers who have relevant training in special needs. It will be particularly important that the class teacher responsible for your child is keen, and that she is made fully aware of your child's needs, method of communicating (especially if he uses signing or an electronic communication system) etc.

We all hope that our children will be able to keep up with their peers and fully participate in the curriculum. However, if your child has severe disabilities or takes a little longer to learn than some others you might have to discuss ways of enabling him to benefit from appropriate education without losing out on activities where he can fully join in with his peers.

The success of placing your child in mainstream schooling will depend on a positive partnership between parents, child, peers, teachers and the Local Education Authority. They should all be working together to ensure that proper planning takes place prior to your child entering school and that you meet regularly throughout his schooling to review progress. Schools are required to appoint a teacher and a governor who have specific responsibility for special educational needs.

Some local authorities have responded to legislation which favours integration by closing special schools but failing to ensure that the mainstream alternatives are properly equipped with trained staff and an appropriate physical environment. Arguments against placing a child in mainstream education include the following:

● Parents fear that their children are more vulnerable than

others and will not be able to cope with the rough and tumble of school life;

- Children with disabilities can become isolated in mainstream schools because they may not be able to keep up with peers;
- Mainstream schools are not properly equipped to deal with special needs;
- Other children might pick out a child who has disabilities for derision and bullying.

Arguments in favour of a mainstream placement include the following:

- If enough parents and children put pressure on local authorities to integrate their children, resources will eventually be channelled appropriately;
- A mainstream environment enables a child with disabilities to grow up to understand and accept the real world in which he lives;
- Mainstream education offers an opportunity for better academic achievement than many special schools are able to;
- A child in mainstream education is more likely to be educated alongside friends from the local community with whom he can develop 'out of school' relationships.
- Mixing disabled and non-disabled pupils will help to break down barriers which might otherwise lead to those without disabilities having negative attitudes and fear around disability when they grow up.

**The success story of an all-ability school in Derbyshire**
Springfield is a school for all in Swadlingcote, Burton on Trent. Pupils ages range from 7–11 years old; 150 pupils are non-disabled and 50 have some kind of special educational need. Some of the pupils have severe disabilities. Springfield has class sizes of less than 20 with two adults in every classroom. All children are taught with their peers in terms of age.

This has been achieved by taking eight teachers who would have been needed for a separate special school for those with special needs and six teachers who would have taught those who are not disabled and dividing the children up amongst the 14 teachers. In addition, the school was able to convince the Local Education Authority of the financial savings which such an arrangement offered – for example, only one head teacher's salary and one school keeper's salary to be provided for and a reduction in all running costs. Because of these savings Springfield was able to negotiate a reimbursement in the form of additional, non-teaching staff to support teachers in the classroom.

Springfield aims to create a school where all children can discover and realise their individual potential, whatever that may be, and where each person's achievements are recognised and valued by their peers.

The benefits of this approach are being felt in the following ways:

- Government inspectors have stated that the needs of children with special educational needs are being met by the school.
- The kind of learning which takes place in an all-ability environment is more relevant to real life.
- Children are able to learn from more conventional role models.
- There has been a reduction in 'ghetto' behaviour. Children with special needs are no longer relegated to their own sector.
- There has emerged an increase in expectations. For example, it has been found that there are children who cannot read who can understand maps.
- A greater width of experience has developed for all. All of the children in the school are able to learn and see what other children need to do in order to learn. For example, some physiotherapy may take place in the classroom. This feeds into the learning curriculum by enabling all children to develop awareness of how the body functions and allows those without disabilities to appreciate the effort put in by their disabled peers.
- There has been a reduction in the use of inappropriate labels.
- Teachers have developed skills they did not know they had by learning from each other's disciplines.
- Additional teaching and non-teaching time is not focused solely on children with special educational needs. This enables those children who find learning particularly easy also to get the benefit of extra input to support their rate of learning.

- Smaller classrooms give teachers a wider range of effective management options in the classroom. Smaller groups can be more appropriately matched.
- There is a lower than average staff turnover because of increased job satisfaction. This leads to smaller recruiting costs.
- Vast sums of money are saved because there is no need to consider sending children to expensive, out of town, special schools as their needs can be met at Springfield.

Since Springfield went all-ability a huge change has taken place in the attitudes of governors and parents. At first there was scepticism of the proposed scheme. Parents of non-disabled children were concerned that the presence of those with special needs would distract the teachers and dilute the effectiveness of teaching. Almost all parents now recognise the value of the shared experience.

At the age of 11, children at Springfield have the option of moving on to a local comprehensive school which is developing a similar philosophy. A local nursery, too, is working hard to develop an under-fives facility based on the same principles.

## Beckford primary school

A three-storey Victorian building in West Hampstead was an unlikely choice for designation to accept children with physical disabilities. A disabled child joined the school in 1991 and the head teacher and governors quickly investigated the possibility of installing a lift and creating ramps. The school now has 450 children with more than 100 children recognised on the Special Educational Needs Register. Class sizes are 30 pupils with two adults in most rooms. The school was funded to appoint a disability co-ordinator and extra non-teaching learning support.

Beckford aims to value all individuals and believes that all children have gifts to share and bring to the school. In this setting the child is seen as a person first and systems are put in place which emphasise both individual strengths and opportunities necessary to maximise their individual potential.

The school favours full-time inclusion rather than the compromise option of part-time 'integration'. The school hopes to share its success with others in and around the borough of

Camden in which it is situated. The experience of Beckford has shown that a school does not have to be very special or different to include all levels of disability in its pupils.

## Special units in mainstream schools

This compromise option is becoming popular in some areas. By having special units within a mainstream setting it is intended that children with disabilities can benefit from social interaction with non-disabled peers and share some lessons with them. Time can also be set aside, within the special unit, for education to focus on the special educational needs which children with disabilities might have.

In practice, the school has to take great care to avoid children in special units becoming isolated in just the same way as they might if removed to a special school. There is still segregation in this practice.

Because special units are only attached to a few mainstream schools it is likely that disabled pupils will still be travelling to schools outside their local community.

## Other options

**Special schools linking with local mainstream schools**
Many special schools form links with local mainstream schools and groups of children can visit between schools for specific sessions. This system is quite often adopted for pupils in special schools who, it is felt, should be slowly integrated into a mainstream setting where they will eventually attend full time.

Unfortunately, it is becoming common for children who attend special schools to be offered a permanent, part-time arrangement with a local mainstream school. Part-time can be as little as 1–3 hours per week and the disabled child is often only invited to participate in non-academic curriculum activities. Members of the inclusive education movement are strongly opposed to these arrangements arguing that they only offer a glimpse into another world for the disabled child and no real participation. It has been contended by the movement that this kind of integration is about as realistic as calling someone 'a little bit pregnant'! You either are or you are not! It can also be extremely disruptive as the disabled child does not know which community they are meant to belong to and which curriculum they are meant to follow.

**Educating your child other than at school** If you are unable to find a suitable school for your child, educating her at home or getting together with other parents who feel similarly disatisfied with the provision on offer may be a real alternative.

There is provision in the 1981 Act for children to be educated 'otherwise' than at school. However, parents must demonstrate that their children are getting an adequate level of education. In certain rare circumstances the local authority might agree that home teaching is in the best interests of the child and provide some teaching assistance at home.

There is a movement of parents who prefer their children (many of whom are not disabled) to be taught at home. More information can be obtained by contacting Education Otherwise – see the list of useful addresses and contacts on page 219.

Another organisation known as the Human Scale Education Movement is keen to promote the idea of education as a lifelong process of development of the whole person helping people to grow, not only in knowledge and skills, but also in health, feeling, judgement, sense of responsibility and creativity. The movement is particularly focused on three initiatives as follows:

- Mini schools and other schemes which allow large scale schools to restructure on a human scale;
- Small schools, especially where the intention is that they should be non-fee paying and have open access; the challenge is to provide a wide curriculum and high adult/ pupil ratio without being 'uneconomical';
- Flexischooling, which encourages schools to combine school with home-based or community-based education.

The Human Scale Education Movement is keen to encourage new initiatives and support parents and teachers working for change in the mainstream.

**Private education** There are a number of private educational establishments with very different philosophies.

Steiner schools have an educational theory which differs from the state education system. They believe in drawing out a child's creative abilities and imagination and do not press children to learn academically until they reach the age of 7. There are a number of Steiner boarding schools which have been set up specifically to cater for children with special educational needs. Some of these schools have enabled children to make enormous progress in social and emotional development in cases where they have suffered deprivation in these areas. Steiner schools use art and music extensively.

If you are interested in Steiner Schools, see the list of useful addresses and contacts (on page 219) to find out more.

Ordinary public schools usually have very specific entrance requirements and you will need to talk to the school in question to find out if it will consider accepting your child and on what basis.

The Montessori system was devised to cater for children with special educational needs. The teaching system is very intensive. Each child's development is individually supported with carefully graded and sequenced learning strategies. Over time the majority of Montessori schools have become mainstream schools and the same issues face children with disabilities entering a Montessori school as those facing children with disabilities entering an ordinary mainstream school. In addition to this the parents will have to find fees.

# 8

# After school – what next?

'What happens next?' is a question which plagues the vast majority of children nearing the time when they leave school and enter the adult world. There is a vast wealth of choice on the surface but, with the increasing demand in the employment market for higher educational qualifications and/or experience these choices are becoming more limited. Choices range from studying for a degree or vocational qualification, going on a youth training scheme if you lack the exam results for higher education, straight into the work place in an unskilled position, unemployment or marriage and raising families (an option still mainly open only to women).

As well as how to earn a living other questions likely to beset a child prior to leaving school include: 'Where will I live when I leave home?' 'Who will I live with?' 'How will my sexual and emotional needs be met?'

Special interests and hobbies are often already developed by the time a child leaves school but not always so, and this can be another area for concern at this important time in every person's life.

Before we go on to look at the particular way in which these issues might affect an emerging adult who has cerebral palsy I would like you to jot down your answers to the following questions. These questions may be hard for you to answer but I urge you to make every effort to do so. Only by taking on such a task can you begin to know what children with disabilities face as they emerge into the adult world.

- Did you leave school with a clear idea of what career you wanted to follow? Please write down details of your experience in this respect.
- Did you follow through with the same career or did your choice change as time went on and how?
- How did the things you learned in school connect with your subsequent life path/career?

- Did you feel confused about your sexuality? In what ways?
- Were there problems in deciding how and when to settle down with the partner of your choice? What sort of problems did you encounter?
- Did you feel afraid about your future security? Why?
- Did you feel the need both to be with your parents and away from them at the same time? Why?

My guess is that you will have found it difficult, if not painful, to look at the issues raised in answering these questions. Add to this a world which assumes that you are virtually incapable of contributing to the job market before you even get a chance to prove yourself, and which does not consider that you can have valid, emotional, sexual or security needs, and consider where this would leave you at the age of 16–21!

I'm going to suggest that we are asking a bit much to expect an emerging adult with disabilities to slot neatly into an often prescribed adult role when most of us left school feeling fairly shaky about our chosen path.

## Options for school leavers who have disabilities

Theoretically, school leavers who have disabilities have broadly similar options to those who do not have disabilities. These fall into the following categories:

**Economic options:**
- Further education/training;
- Employment (full-time or part-time);
- Unemployment;
- Home-based activities (such as becoming a housewife).

**Living situation options:**
- Staying at home with parents;
- Settling down with a partner;
- Living independently in your own home;
- Living in a community setting.

**Social options:**
- Finding/having a peer group to share entertainment with;
- Expanding and building on non-work interests (hobbies etc.);

- Broadening your solitary entertainment (reading, listening to music, watching television etc.);
- Having sexual experiences.

It is impossible to generalise about the ways in which these options will present different obstacles for young adults who have cerebral palsy. It is important to remember that they are all likely to *be* obstacles in some way or another for anyone. The young adult with CP is, however, likely to have extra hurdles to leap over while finding their way into adult life and there are a number of institutions and services which might be able to help make the passage easier.

## Further education

All young people have a legal right to education until their 19th birthday. Many stay on at school, transfer to another school or enter a local or residential college.

If your child has a statement of special educational needs this should be re-assessed when he is 14 years old with preliminary discussion of future plans. The head teacher at your child's school should be approached about this.

The most traditional further education paths at the age of 16 are the following:

- To move from secondary school to a sixth form centre (unless the secondary school has its own sixth form) so that study can begin for advanced examinations which would enable entrance to university.
- Attendance at an appropriate institution for training in technical and vocational skills. The two most common courses are: The Certificate of pre-Vocational Education (CPVE) and the Technical and Vocational Education Initiative (TVEI). These courses usually run from the age of 14 up to 18.

It is quite common for children who are in special schools to stay on at school after they are 16 years old. This is often found beneficial particularly to pupils who may have had interruptions in their education for health reasons.

In some areas pupils can attend 'link courses' at a local further education college while they are still attending school for one or two days per week. Link courses are particularly useful for students who are considered to have moderate learning difficulties.

There are assessment centres which are intended to help people with disabilities to find out what their capabilities are and make realistic plans for the future. The two main types of assessment centre are as follows:

- Those which offer a comprehensive assessment of a young person's abilities and skills with courses offered for remedial education, vocational training, work experience and training in independence and mobility (these should be available through your Social Services Department or the Local Education Authority). The Queen Elizabeth Foundation for the Disabled and the Royal National Institute for the Blind also offer comprehensive assessment facilities (see the list of contacts and further addresses on pages 219–231). The Queen Elizabeth Foundation also produces a directory of opportunities for school leavers, a copy of which should be available at your local careers office or from the foundation itself.
- Those which aim to help young people with disabilities to decide on appropriate employment training or work. These assessment centres are known as Employment Rehabilitation Centres and are offered by the Training Agency which is part of the Department of Employment. Your local job centre should have details.

There are a number of further education institutes which specialise in offering further education for people who have disabilities. Many of these are residential and involve the student in studying away from home. Voluntary organisations, including Scope, MENCAP, the RNIB and RNID run residential colleges for disabled students. In most cases students will be paid for by their Local Education Authority.

In addition, a number of mainstream colleges and universities offer (usually limited) facilities to aid independence in a mainstream setting. The approach is not always as enabling as it may at first appear.

The disabled teenager is likely to encounter extra obstacles and be required to put in much more effort than a non-disabled peer just to be able to go to a further educational establishment. Special arrangements may have to be made for examinations (which you need to know about and apply for in advance). Is the education worth the physical obstacles of access and transport difficulties? An example of the piecemeal way in which integration is attempted was demonstrated by one London college which carefully geared up its computer department for wheelchair access and was disappointed to find that the opportunity was not taken up by any wheelchair users. The college had failed to take account of the transport difficulties a disabled student might have, and there were no disabled toilets in the building.

The choice between specialised or mainstream further education is likely to be heavily influenced by how much social independence has been achieved by the student. Specialist institutions will offer courses on independent living and social skills as well as vocational or academic training. However, there have been criticisms made that some specialist institutions put too much emphasis on social skills and not enough on academic skills.

The National Bureau for Handicapped Students has a range of useful literature. The National Union of Students produces guides on halls of residence, and grants and awards.

The training division of the Manpower Services Commission has four residential training centres which cater for the further educational needs of adults with a wide range of severity of disability.

## The Open University

The Open University offers home-based further education with special facilities for students with disabilities. It offers a wide range of courses which can either lead to the obtaining of a full degree or certificates which will enhance work opportunities. The system is designed to cater for students who are not able to study full-time and you can therefore spread your degree course over a number of years whilst building up skills and confidence in other areas or undertaking employment.

If you are continuing in education your benefits should not be disrupted unless you are attending residential establishments, in which case your Attendance Allowance might be affected. You might only be able to claim Attendance Allowance for the periods you are actually at home. A student may qualify for an Educational Maintenance Allowance if their parents' income is very low.

# Finding work

In employment, as in every other aspect of life, the disabled person has the added disadvantage of negative attitudes to contend with. In 1986 a study into discrimination in employment against people with disabilities was commissioned by Scope and undertaken by Eileen Fry. The method employed was very simple. Employers' responses to two (fictitious) letters of application, which differed only in that one was from a disabled applicant and the other was not, were analysed. In 41 per cent of cases disabled applicants received a negative response while non-disabled applicants received a positive one. In only 3 per cent of cases was the reverse true. There were examples in the study of non-disabled people being asked to interview while disabled applicants with exactly the same qualifications were not. In some cases disabled applicants were informed that the position had been filled while the non-disabled applicant was invited to interview.

There are a number of schemes to help people with disabilities to get an ordinary job. Job centres employ Disablement Resettlement Officers who are taught to discuss alternatives and the careers service employs Specialist Careers Officers.

There are a number of employment services available to people with disabilities.

## *The Manpower Services Commission (MSC)*

This was set up under the Employment and Training Act 1973. Its employment division runs the network of local employment offices and job centres. The Disablement Resettlement Officer service is included in this as well as the administration of sheltered employment for the disabled. The Local Authority Careers Service is also administered under the MSC. All careers officers have a duty to assist young disabled people.

The local employment office or job centre can provide a disabled person with registration. This can be helpful in finding employment as large firms are required, by law, to employ a quota of persons who are registered disabled.

The three criteria for registration are:

- That the applicant is substantially handicapped in finding and keeping suitable employment;
- That the disability is likely to last for at least 12 months;

- That the applicant wants a job and has a reasonable chance of obtaining and keeping one.

The Employment Division of the MSC runs a network of 27 employment rehabilitation centres which offer courses aimed at restoring physical capacity and confidence and assessing ability as well as giving advice about the type of work most likely to offer permanent employment.

## Self-employment

Self-employment is becoming an increasingly popular way to earn a living and may have particular attractions for the adult who has disabilities in that the problems of transport and availability of disabled facilities (such as toilets) are avoided. However, working for yourself often involves long hours and has the disadvantage that workplace training opportunities are not available. In addition to this the self-employed person has to take responsibility for his own tax and National Insurance payments.

Self-employed people are not eligible for Statutory Sick Pay or Maternity Pay. If they have paid the requisite number of Class II National Insurance Payments, however, they should be eligible for Statutory Sickness Benefit (1996 rates, £47.35 per week), or, if having a baby, for 18 weeks Maternity Allowance (1996 rates, £54.55 per week). The leaflets *FB 28 Sick or Disabled?* and *FB 8 Babies and Benefits*, both available from your local Social Services Department, Citizens' Advice Bureau or Post Office, will give you more information.

Advice on self-employment can be sought from the 'Small Firms Service' provided by the Department of Industry.

## Incentives for businesses to employ people with disabilities

There are a number of incentives available to encourage firms to employ people with disabilities.

- The MSC can provide grants to employers for adaptation of their buildings to accommodate the needs of disabled employees.
- Large firms are legally obliged to employ a quota of people who are registered disabled.

- Assistance is available to employees who are not able to use public transport to get to and from work. Application should be made to the Disablement Resettlement Officer for your area.
- Aids and equipment to enable disabled individuals to carry out their job may be available free or for loan through the Disablement Resettlement Officer.
- The Job Introduction Scheme enables the MSC to make a weekly grant to employers who engage a selected disabled person for a trial period of up to 13 weeks. This scheme is meant to encourage employers to allow the disabled person to prove her ability to perform a particular job.

## CSV in the workplace

Community Service Volunteers also run a scheme whereby a volunteer can accompany a person with a disability to work and carry out basic tasks (such as typing and filing) for him to enable him to carry out his job.

## Considerations for people with disabilities in mainstream employment

There are a wide variety of positions which can be filled by people with even severe disabilities provided that access to the place of employment is arranged and specialist equipment available where necessary.

The advent of computer technology has made the office environment much more accessible for people with disabilities and there is a wide range of courses available to enable people with disabilities to develop their computer skills. In addition, there are many computer accessories now available which can enable even a severely disabled person with restricted limb movement to manage a computer system competently. Telephone systems can be adapted for those who might have difficulty with an ordinary telephone mouthpiece.

Employers may be surprised to find how efficient and able an employee with disabilities can be as their motivation to achieve and to prove themselves is likely to be high.

One of the cleanest and most efficient office environments I have had contact with was the Islington Disablement Association who I had occasion to visit for advice on benefits as well as for help with research for this publication. There is a fairly high percentage of employees who have disabilities. I was given coffee while I waited, all my queries were answered (or appropriate advice given on where to go for more information) and the organisation was quick to send me fairly bulky photocopied information which I requested. I came away feeling that employees who have reservations about taking on people with disabilities would learn a lot from a visit here and perhaps clear away some of their prejudice.

It is noticeable that the organisations who lead the way in having good employment practices are those which actually cater for the needs of people with disabilities. Even in these organisations, however, there are very few people with disabilities who have senior positions. Basically this comes back to education. Unless students with disabilities are given a real opportunity to gain qualifications and appropriate training there will always be an inequality in higher management positions. The only way to achieve this is to offer the disabled student the same options as those who are not disabled and to ensure that the facilities are in place to allow access to educational establishments. Although there is a lack of funding in this area there is also a lack of awareness amongst employers and educators regarding the needs of people with disabilities and, often, a lack of commitment to taking the necessary steps to improve people's opportunities.

All of this contributes to high unemployment among disabled people, and the low average wage (an estimated 40 per cent of people with disabilities have incomes which are below the poverty line, according to The Report of the London Housing Enquiry) among those fortunate enough to gain employment.

## Sheltered work

A small number of people are so severely disabled that they are unable to cope with employment under normal conditions although they are able to carry out productive work with appropriate support. The Disablement Resettlement Office can offer advice in such situations. Three sources for access to this type of work are Remploy, local authorities and voluntary organisations.

**Remploy** This is a Government-supported company set up to provide employment for severely disabled men and women who are unable to obtain or retain work in open industry. A disabled person must register with the MSC in order to pursue work with Remploy.

**Local authorities**   Local authorities run a number of workshops where a disabled person can obtain sheltered work for which she will receive proper wages and pay tax and gain insurance benefits.

**Voluntary organisations**   The Queen Elizabeth Foundation for the disabled is an example. Sheltered Industrial Groups (SIGs) offer opportunities for people with disabilities to work alongside those who do not have disabilities in an ordinary working environment with special supervisory support. SIGs opportunities are particularly useful in less populated areas where the setting up of workshops is not feasible.

## Day centres

Local authorities run day centres which are establishments open daily and offering recreational activities and assistance with improving independence for people whose disabilities are of sufficient severity to prevent them from working. Day centre workers are employed to facilitate activities and there are commonly group activities available on a regular basis. From my own experience of working in a day centre, examples of the kinds of activity which used to be available include: arts and crafts, music, printing, reality orientation for elderly people with Alzheimer's disease, practice with domestic tasks, reading groups, newsletter production and similar activities. I remember one gentleman who was fairly elderly and immobile due to motor neurone disease but who had an extremely agile mind discovering an ability to invent crossword puzzles through his involvement in the newsletter we produced on a monthly basis. Planning the monthly crossword helped to restore his confidence and sense of purpose. On the other hand I also remember a teenage boy with severe cerebral palsy who attended the centre being left to sit in his wheelchair for long periods of time without stimulation. It is well worth checking out the extent of the staff's understanding of cerebral palsy and what activities they would propose to offer before recommending this option to an adult who has CP.

Social Services can advise on day centres in the locality.

# Relationships and sexuality

Forming close relationships can pose problems for people who have physical disabilities. In the first instance the problems may be those experienced by all young people growing up and becoming aware of their sexuality. Puberty is confusing for most adolescents and, over the years, the education system has taken on board the need to prepare young people for adulthood in providing sex education (albeit in an often clinical way).

However, young people with disabilities are often regarded as asexual beings. It is often assumed that they will be barred from an active sexual life and parents and educationalists often fail to recognise that the feelings and needs of an adolescent with disabilities are likely to be exactly the same as the non-disabled adolescent. In addition to this, the disabled adolescent may well develop complexes around issues of sexuality as part of a general pattern of low self-esteem, lack of confidence and lack of information.

It is *absolutely wrong* to assume that someone who has cerebral palsy has no sexual feelings or that they cannot enjoy a fulfilling sex life. It may be that certain positions are awkward and that they will need to discover ways to obtain full sexual enjoyment which take account of whatever physical difficulties they experience but sexual enjoyment is as much a right as any other equal opportunity issue facing an adult with disabilities.

There is an emergence of more literature on sex and disability as well as a number of organisations which aim specifically to support people with disabilities in forming meaningful relationships and having a satisfying sex life. ASBAH have joined forces with The Spastics Society to produce a very useful book for adolescents called *Sex for Young People with Spina Bifida and Cerebral Palsy*. Other publications include *Life Together* by Inger Nordqvist, *Entitled to Love: The Sexual and Emotional Needs of the Handicapped* by Dr Wendy Greengross and *Handicapped Married Couples* by Michael and Ann Craft (see also the further reading list on page 232).

Organisations worth contacting include: Disdate (a penfriend and dating agency), The Outsiders Club (formed to bring together people who have become emotionally stranded and to help each other to find partners, friendship and love), SPOD (Association to aid the sexual and personal relationships of the disabled), Gemma (an organisation for disabled and non-disabled lesbians which aims to lessen isolation of those whose disability may hinder them from forming relationships and pursuing lesbian relationships) and the Gay Men's Disabled Group (which aims to provide support to gay men who have disabilities and to bring them together with gay men who do not have disabilities). The list of contacts and useful addresses on pages 219–231 gives further information.


## Sport and leisure

Where they are satisfied there is a real need, local authorities are empowered by the Chronically Sick and Disabled Persons Act 1970 to help disabled people who are resident in their area to enjoy a wide range of recreational activities. This includes, for example, help to obtain radio and television sets and to attend lectures, games, outings and other leisure pursuits. Arrangements differ from one local authority to another so you need to contact your own local authority for further information. Information is also available from the British Sports Association for the Disabled which has locally based representatives who can advise on facilities in your area.

There are numerous organisations and publications which concentrate on specific sport or leisure activities for people with disabilities. Please see the lists of useful contacts and addresses, and further reading for more information.

# 9

# Legal rights and benefits

## Legislation

This section outlines much of the relevant legislation which has been put in place to safeguard the rights of people with disabilities and to make provision for them to receive appropriate services.

### Disability in general

**The National Assistance Act 1948**   This Act defines the term 'disabled', as describing people who are 'blind, deaf or dumb, and other persons who are substantially and permanently handicapped by illness, injury or congenital deformity or who are suffering from a mental disorder within the meaning of the Mental Health Act'.

Part III of this Act places a duty on local authorities to provide residential care and powers and duties to provide welfare services for disabled people.

**The Mental Health Act 1983**   This Act describes individuals as suffering from a mental disorder if they have a mental illness, arrested or incomplete development of mind, psychopathic disorder and any other disorder or disability of mind.

**The Chronically Sick and Disabled Persons Act 1970**   Under Section 1 of this Act, local authorities must:

- Take steps to inform themselves of the numbers and needs of disabled persons in their area;
- Publish information as to the services they provide under the 1948 National Assistance Act;
- Ensure that disabled persons are informed of any available services which in the opinion of the authority are relevant to their needs.

Under Section 2 of this Act, the local authority is duty bound to meet the needs of disabled residents as set out below:

- Provision of practical assistance for that person in their home;
- Provision, or assistance to that person in obtaining wireless, television, library or similar recreational activities;
- Provision for that person of lectures, games, outings or other recreational facilities outside the home or assistance in taking advantage of educational facilities available to him;
- Provision or assistance with travel for the purpose of participating in any activity which is provided by the local authority as a service under the 1948 National Assistance Act;
- The provision of assistance in arranging for the carrying out of any adaptations to the home or provision of additional facilities designed to secure his greater safety, comfort or convenience;
- Facilitating the taking of holidays by that person, whether at holiday homes or otherwise and whether provided under arrangements made by the authority or otherwise;
- The provision of meals for that person whether in his home or elsewhere;
- The provision for that person of, or assistance to obtain, a telephone and any special equipment necessary to enable him to use the telephone.

Section 3 requires local authorities to consider the special housing needs of the chronically sick and disabled.

Sections 4, 5, 6, 8, 8a and 8b require that, in providing buildings open to the public, provision must be made for the needs of disabled visitors in internal and external access, parking and lavatories. There is a rider within these sections that all such provision is only required 'in as far as it is, in the circumstances, practical and reasonable'.

Section 7 provides for the publicising of amenities outlined in the preceding sections.

Sectons 9–15 and 23 provide for disabled persons (or those experienced in working with disabled persons) to serve on advisory bodies and local authority committees wherever possible.

Section 16 requires the National Advisory Council of Disabled Persons to provide for the training of those who train or find employment for disabled people.

Sections 17 and 18 require that disabled people under the age of 65 should not be cared for in old people's homes.

Section 20 provides for wheelchairs to be used on footpaths and pavements without the need to carry lights.

Secton 21 provides for the issue of orange badges by local authorities to help with disabled people's parking needs.

**The Local Authorities Social Services Act 1970** This Act requires local authorities to establish social services committees to deal with (among other things):

* Provision of residential accommodation for the elderly and infirm;
* Welfare of persons who are disabled under the National Assistance Act 1948;
* Provision of facilities to enable disabled persons to be employed or work under special conditions;
* Prevention of illness and care and after-care of the sick;
* Provision of home help and laundry facilities for certain households;
* Promotion of welfare of old people;
* Financial and other assistance to voluntary organisations;
* Obtaining information and publishing information as to the existence of certain welfare services;
* Provision of welfare services.

**Local Government Act 1972** This Act provides for consultation by district councils with respect to the nature and extent of the accommodation needed for people who, because of infirmity or disability, need accommodation of a special character.

**The National Health Services Act 1977** Section 5 allows the Secretary of State to provide invalid carriages. (In practice no new invalid carriages are being issued).

Section 8 lays a duty on local social services to provide home help on a scale adequate for the needs of their area in a variety of circumstances. It also gives such authorities the power to arrange for the provision of laundry facilities for which the local authority is entitled to recover a charge having regard to the means of the beneficiaries.

**Disabled Persons Act 1981** Section 1 inserts a new section into the Highway Act 1980 requiring statutory authorities responsible for highways to consider the needs of disabled or blind people when carrying out, in a street, work which impedes their mobility. It also requires the authority to have regard to the needs of disabled people when considering the provision of ramps at appropriate places between highways and footways.

Section 2 amends the Road Traffic Regulations Act 1967 by making the infringement of a disabled parking space illegal. It also makes wrongful use of an orange badge illegal.

Section 3 inserts new Sections 29A and B into the Town and Country Planning Act 1971 concerning the granting of planning permission in respect of premises covered by sections 4–8A of the Chronically Sick and Disabled Persons Act 1970 and requires the British Standards Institute to draw attention to the relevant provisions of that Act.

Section 4 amends Section 20 of the Local Government Act 1976 to ensure that when a notice is served to provide, maintain, keep clean or make available 'sanitary appliances' at a place of entertainment, attention is drawn to Sections 6 and 7 of the Chronically Sick and Disabled Persons Act 1970, and to the British Standards Institute Code of Practice (Access for the Disabled to Buildings).

Section 5 provides a new Section 7 to the Chronically Sick and Disabled Persons Act 1970.

Section 6 further amends the Chronically Sick and Disabled Persons Act by deleting (under Sections 4, 5, 6, 8 and 8a) the words 'in so far as it is in the circumstances practical and reasonable' to the requirement of 'appropriate provision' in accordance with the British Standards Code of Practice.

Section 7 inserts Section 8B into the Chronically Sick and Disabled Persons Act 1970.

**The Disabled Persons Act 1986**  This Act received Royal Assent on the 8th July 1986 and a phased implementation was agreed on account of the high resourcing implications of the Act. At the time of writing, there are still sections of the Act which are due to be implemented and there is a lobby within the disabled community for implementation to be speeded up.

Section 1 provides for the appointment of an 'authorised representative' for people with disabilities. This is defined as someone appointed by or on behalf of a disabled person to act as his 'advocate'. *No date has been fixed for implementation.*

Section 2 requires local authorities to allow the repesentative to act on the disabled person's behalf in connection with the provision of any social services. There is scope within this section for representation, after consultation with the Secretary of State, to extend to the Health Authorities. *No date has been fixed for implementation.*

Section 3 requires local authorities to allow disabled people to make representation about their needs before an assessment takes place and gives them the right to ask for a review of any decision. *No date has been fixed for implementation.*

Section 4 confirms that local authorities must assess the needs of a disabled person for any of the services listed in the Chronically Sick and Disabled Persons Act 1970 if asked to do so by the person, his representative or carer. *This was implemented in April 1987 except regarding the abilities of carers.*

Section 5 requires Local Education Authorities to seek information from Social Services (at the first annual review after the child's fourteenth birthday) as to whether a child with a statement under the Education Act 1981 is disabled. The Education Authority must inform Social Services eight months before the person's presumed date of leaving school or further education. Social Services must undertake an assessment within five months of receiving notification unless the person asks them not to do so. *Implemented February 1988.*

Section 7 refers to anyone who has been an in-patient in a hospital for a continuous period of six months or more for a 'mental disorder' and establishes the principle of co-operation between health and local authorities.

Hospital managers must inform the District Health Authority, the local authority where a person intends to live, and the Local Education Authority of the date of discharge from hospital if the person is under 19 years old.

Before the discharge date the District Health Authority must make an arrangement for an assessment of need to be carried out. This section ensures that long-stay patients are not suddenly discharged without assessment and services being arranged beforehand. *No date has been fixed for implementation.*

Section 8 places a duty on the local authority to take account of the needs of carers (defined as people other than paid staff, who are providing a substantial amount of care for a disabled person). *Implemented April 1987.*

Section 9 requires Social Services Departments to inform disabled people who are already receiving social services, of relevant services provided by the local authority, or any other authority or organisation on which they have information. *Implemented April 1987.*

Section 10 provides for the co-option to committees of people representing the interests of disabled people. Specifically it provides that appropriate organisations should be consulted before appointment or co-option is made. *Implemented April 1987.*

Section 11 requires the Secretary of State to produce an annual report to Parliament on the development of community services for mentally ill or mentally handicapped people, the number of people receiving in-patient treatment for mental illness or mental handicap and other information he considers appropriate. This Section enables some monitoring of the progress of community care policies for people with mental illness and/or mental handicaps. *No date fixed for implementation.*

**The Community Care Act 1991**   This is dealt with more fully in Chapter 6, pages 115–145.

**Disability Discrimination Act 1995**   This is normally referred to as the DDA and is being introduced gradually with many disability groups dissatisfied with its powers. One of the more immediate measures of DDA is to make it unlawful for car insurance companies to load higher premiums onto disabled drivers, but other aspects of the Act will take longer to implement. For example, education is still not being considered. Some aspects of DDA are vague e.g. when it says that the Act will make it unlawful to refuse to serve a disabled customer 'unless justified'!

The disability rights movement are very unhappy about this Act which has been introduced in place of a very carefully thought out draft that they themselves produced giving detailed planning and timescales to enable full inclusion into society. They contend that it does very little to increase the rights of disabled people to a full place in society. For more information about this Act contact Disability on the Agenda, Freepost, Bristol, BS38 7DE.

## Education

The law relating to education has been largely outlined in Chapter 7, but the key acts are summarised briefly below:

**Education Act 1944**   This Act requires that sufficient schooling and educational facilities are made available by Local Education Authorities to meet the need in their area with a legal obligation to provide for the special education needs of pupils up to the age of 18 by regular attendance at school or otherwise.

**Education Act 1953**   Empowers local authorities, with approval from the Secretary of State, to arrange for the provision of primary or secondary school education for pupils to be at non-maintained schools with fees paid in certain circumstances:

- Where, because of shortage of alternatives or the special educational needs of the child, the authority cannot directly provide for his education;
- Where the authority is satisfied that the pupil has special educational needs and that it is expedient in his interests that the required special educational need should be made for the pupil at a school not maintained by the Education Authority.

**Education (Handicapped Children) Act 1970**   Provided for the discontinuance of classifying handicapped children as being unsuitable for education at school.

**Education Act 1980**   Section 8 provides for information to be provided by Local Education Authorities in relation to special education. In particular it calls for:

- The identification and assessment of children with special educational needs and the involving of parents in that process;
- The provision made in all schools maintained by them for pupils with special educational needs;
- Special educational provision otherwise than at school;
- The authorities' arrangements and policies regarding non-maintained schools;
- Arrangements being made in respect of transport;
- The arrangements for parents to obtain advice and further information.

This Act provides that information should be made available in two ways: firstly, by copies being available to parents without charge on request; and secondly, by copies being available to parents for reference at every school maintained by the state and in public libraries in the area of that authority.

**Education Act 1981**   This Act was a direct response to the Warnock Report (1978, *Special Needs in Education*) which called for greater integration opportunities into mainstream schools for pupils with special educational needs. The implications of this Act for carers and their children who have disabilities was examined in more detail in Chapter 7.

**Education Act 1993 and Code of Practice 1994**   This act has tightened up the responsibility of Local Education Authorities to carry out their duties within certain time limits. It also offers the possibility of more independent appeal bodies and strengthens the role of pupils and parents in determining children's educational futures. Unfortunately the Act does not give parents the absolute right to choose where their children are educated. More details are contained in Chapter 7.

**The Children's Act 1989**   This Act marks a very significant reform of the law relating to all children, and in particular imposes duties on local authorities to provide assistance and services for children 'in need'.

Section 17 (1) of the Act places a duty on every local authority to:

- Safeguard and promote the welfare of children within their area who are in need; and
- So far as it is consistent with their duty, to promote the upbringing of such children by their families, by providing a large level of services appropriate to those children's needs.

These duties are to be carried out as follows:

- The local authority should publish information about services and take reasonable steps to ensure that those who might benefit from these services gain access to them.
- By keeping a register of disabled children within their area.
- Where a child appears in need his needs may be assessed under this Act at the same time as any assessment under

The Chronically Sick and Disabled Persons Act and The Education Act 1981.

- The local authority should provide services designed to minimise the effect on disabled children within their area of their disabilities; and give such children the opportunity to lead lives which are as normal as possible.
- The authority should also make provision for children in need of the following services: advice, guidance and counselling; occupation, social, cultural or recreational activities; home help (possibly including laundry facilities); facilities for travelling to and from home to take advantage of each service; and assistance to enable child and family to have a holiday.

Another important provision is that of day care for pre-school children and the provision of supervised activities as is appropriate, outside school hours or during school holidays, for children in need.

If the local authority fails to provide an adequate service, under Section 26 of the Act local authorities must establish a procedure for considering representations (including complaints) made by a parent of a child in need.

## Employment

**Disabled Persons (Employment) Act 1944** This Act defines a 'disabled person' as one who, 'on account of injury, disease (including a physical or mental condition arising from imperfect development of any organ), or congenital deformity, is substantially handicapped in obtaining or keeping employment, of a kind which apart from that injury, disease or deformity would be suited to his age, experience and qualifications'.

The main provisions of the Act are as follows:

- To set up a register of 'disabled persons' with the aim of ensuring that the fact that an individual's name is on the register will afford reasonable assurance of his being a person capable of entering into and keeping employment, or of undertaking work on his own account.
- An employer who normally has a workforce of more than 20 must give employment to a quota of registered disabled persons (currently 3 per cent).

- Certain categories of employment may be reserved for disabled persons at the discretion of the Secretary of State. This is rarely used in practice. Car park attendants and lift attendants may be covered by this.
- The Secretary of State may provide special facilities for the employment of persons so seriously disabled as to be unable to obtain normal employment or to sustain a business of their own in competition with able bodied people.

**Disabled Persons (Employment) Act 1958**   This Act allows a registered disabled person to have his name removed from the register on written request. It also imposes a duty on local authorities to provide 'sheltered' employment for registered disabled persons.

**Employment and Training Act 1973**   This Act established the Manpower Services Commission which is charged with the duty to make arrangements it considers appropriate to assist persons to select, transfer, obtain and retain employment suitable for their ages and capacities.

**The Companies (Employment of Disabled Persons) Regulations 1980**   These regulations require every directors' report of a company to whom the regulations apply (those with more than 250 employees) to contain a statement describing policies for giving fair consideration to applications for employment from disabled people, for continuing the employment of, and arranging appropriate training for, employees who become disabled during the period they are employed by the company and otherwise for the training, career development and promotion of disabled persons employed by the company.

## Mobility

**The Road Traffic Act 1972**   This Act sets out the conditions for obtaining a licence to drive.

Section 87/87A sets out circumstances where the power to refuse a licence is allowed for certain disabilities as follows:

- Epilepsy;
- Severe subnormality or mental deficiency;
- Liability to sudden attack of giddiness resulting from heart defect or any other cause;

- Inability to read in good daylight;
- Any other disability likely to be a source of danger to the public.

Applicants for licences are under a legal obligation to declare a disability except in the case of temporary disability (those likely to last three months or less).

There are exceptions to the refusal to withhold a licence as outlined below:

- Where a disability is of a non-progressive nature and consists solely of the absence, loss or deformity of one or more limbs.
- Epilepsy which is appropriately controlled. Under this clause the applicant must demonstrate that he has not had an epileptic fit for over two years and that the driving of a vehicle is not likely to be a source of danger to the public.
- A disorder or defect of the heart which is under control with a pacemaker. The applicant must satisfy the conditions that his driving is not likely to be a source of danger to the public and he has made adequate arrangements to receive regular medical supervision.

Under the EEC Directive 80/1263 EC, Article 6, new driving licences can be granted only to those who pass a practical and theoretical test and who meet certain medical standards.

A vehicle constructed or adapted for use for the carriage of one person, being a person suffering from some physical defect or disability, may be driven without a licence. This vehicle is called an invalid carriage and must not exceed 250 lb laden, must not be capable of exceeding four miles per hour, must have brakes which comply with current regulations and must have front and rear lights and rear reflectors.

## Motor Vehicles (Wearing of Seat Belts) Regulations 1982
This law governs the use of seat belts. People with disabilities are exempt from this only if they hold a statutory form of certificate, signed by a registered medical practitioner, to the effect that it is inadvisable on medical grounds for the holder to wear a seat belt.

## The Disabled Persons (Badge for Motor Vehicles) Regulations 1982 This regulates the use of the Orange Badge

scheme. This scheme is designed to help severely disabled people with mobility and parking problems by allowing them special privileges in the form of parking concessions. Drivers with blind passengers, or who carry children with severe disabilities may also benefit from the scheme.

Eligibility is determined by one or more of the following factors:

- Receipt of Mobility Allowance;
- Blind passengers;
- Use of vehicles supplied by government departments or receipt of grants towards the applicant's own vehicle.
- Having a permanent and substantial disability which makes the person unable to walk, or to have very considerable difficulty in walking.

**Transport Act 1968**   This Act empowers local authorities to make travel concessions for men over 65, women over 60, people so blind as to be unable to perform any work for which sight is essential and people suffering from any disability or injury which, in the opinion of the local authority, seriously impairs their ability to walk.

## Suing the local Health Authority for medical negligence which caused cerebral palsy

No health professional will be deliberately negligent and you may feel reluctant to pursue a claim against your local Health Authority either because you feel that they did not intend any harm to your child or because you do not realise that negligence was involved. However, Health Authorities are heavily insured against such claims and you are entitled to make a claim if there is any possibility that what happened to your child could have been avoided by more vigilant health care. There is almost always this possibility even though, at the end of the day, you might not win the case.

Once negligence (however slight) is established the award of money is made on the basis of the severity of the child's disability and not on the extent of the negligence.

Negligence can mean many different things. It might come down to failure on the part of the medical team servicing your birth sufficiently to monitor the process. In some cases, negligence may be evident in the antenatal care. For example, your hospital or GP may fail to act on disturbing signs which become apparent during the progress of the pregnancy. However, it is essential to prove that any negligence *directly* caused the damage. If the child would have been disabled anyway (for example due to congenital factors) then, even if the health professionals were negligent, you may not have a compensation entitlement.

The only way to establish whether you are likely to have a case is to test it out with a solicitor. The organisation Action for Victims of Medical Abuse (AVMA) is trained in assessment of medical negligence and will be able to advise you as to whether you have a case which is worth pursuing. If you do decide to pursue a case AVMA can provide you with the legal advice, back up and representation usually by finding you an appropriately qualified solicitor who will take on your case.

The recent legal change in this area is of great help to parents pursuing claims of medical negligence. It is now standard practice for children who are pursuing claims (even if the claim is being pursued by parents on their behalf) to be assessed for legal aid on the basis of their own incomes and not that of their parents. This has opened the way for many families to pursue claims whereas they previously would not have been able to afford the legal fees.

If medical negligence is proved you will not automatically receive a large sum of money to spend on your child. The needs of your child will be closely scrutinised and assessed. The money awarded can either be held in a trust fund to which you must apply for financial assistance, or administered by a nominated carer. It is very important, therefore, that you have good documented evidence of your child's current and likely future needs to enable you to gain access to the money for your child's benefit.

## Benefits

This section is not a fully comprehensive guide of all state benefits. It concentrates on benefits which are likely to be applicable to people who have cerebral palsy.

For a full outline of benefits you may be entitled to you are strongly advised to obtain a copy of the *Disability Rights Handbook* produced by The Disability Alliance and updated annually. What follows is a brief outline of benefits to which you may be entitled.

Some benefits are available in the form of financial assistance; others may be provision of equipment or certain entitlements (such as cheap or free travel passes).

## Financial aid

**Recent and forthcoming changes**   The benefit system for people with disabilities is currently in the process of change. The new system came into effect from the 1st April 1992. Under the old system, Attendance Allowance and Mobility Allowance were separate benefits and individuals had to be assessed separately for each. Under the new system these two allowances will be amalgamated into a new benefit called the Disability Living Allowance. In addition a further benefit, Disability Working Allowance, is being introduced. This is a means-tested benefit which works in a similar way to Family Credit. The process for assessing families to receive benefit and for adjudication is also changed under the new benefit system.

**The Disability Living Allowance**   This benefit replaces the old Attendance Allowance and Mobility Allowance. However, there are two components to the new allowance which are similar to the benefit being replaced. The first component (replacing Attendance Allowance) is the 'care component'. The second component (replacing Mobility Allowance) is the 'mobility component'. There are three rates of pay for the care component and two rates of pay for the mobility component.

**The care component**   There is no lower age limit on applications for this component. People who are 65 or over are only eligible to apply for one of the two higher care components.

To qualify for the lowest rate of the care component the applicant must be severely disabled, physically or mentally, to the extent that:

- He requires in connection with his bodily functions, attention from another person for a significant portion of the day (whether during a single period or a number of periods); or
- He cannot prepare a cooked meal for himself if he has all the ingredients.

To qualify for the middle rate of the care component the applicant's disability should be so severe that:

- He requires frequent attention throughout the day in connection with his bodily functions (such as going to the toilet, washing or eating); or
- He needs continual supervision throughout the day in order to avoid substantial danger to himself or others.

Alternative conditions which can be met to qualify for the middle rate are as follows:

- The person requires from another person prolonged or repeated attention in connection with his bodily functions; or
- In order to avoid substantial danger to himself and others, the person requires 'another person to be awake for a prolonged period or at frequent intervals for the purpose of watching over' him.

To qualify for the highest rate of the care component claimants must satisfy *either* of the two conditions from each of the alternative sets of conditions outlined for the middle rate.

**The mobility component** This component can only be claimed by children over the age of 5 and adults under the age of 65. People may only claim the mobility component after their 65th birthday if they are not aged more than 66, and they can prove that they would have been eligible before their 65th birthday.

There are two components to this allowance. To qualify for the highest rate, the individual must be:

- On account of physical disablement, mental handicap, severe learning difficulties or very challenging behaviour either unable or virtually unable to walk. (This does not apply to people who are mentally ill). This should include account of the exertion required to walk and consideration for people who are deaf and blind.

To qualify for the lower rate you must be:

- Able to walk but so severely disabled physically or mentally that to take advantage of the faculty out of doors you require guidance or supervision from another person most of the time.

Claimants under the age of 16 for either the mobility or the care component must also show that:

- They require more guidance or supervision from another person than persons of their age in normal physical and mental health would require; or that
- Persons of their age in normal physical and mental health would not require such guidance or supervision.

People claiming the Disability Living Allowance must be resident in the United Kingdom for six out of twelve months prior to award. In addition, there is a rule (under the old Attendance Allowance regulations) that they should not be in residential accommodation, which is financed by a local authority, for more than 28 days. The 28 days are calculated by adding together any stays in such residential accommodation which occur within 28 days of each other. If the 28 days are used up, claimants will not be able to claim for any whole days spent in residential care but they will be able to get it for any day at home including the days on which they go into and leave the residential care home. Once they have spent a continuous period of more than 28 days at home, they are entitled to a new allocation of 28 days on which the component can be paid while they are away from home.

To qualify for either component there is a three month waiting or qualifying period before an award will be made. It is also likely that payments will only be made to people who are expected to have relevant care needs or mobility restrictions for nine months or more following the award.

There is no facility for claimants to backdate their claims. You are only eligible from the date you apply (adding on the prescribed waiting period).

It is not yet clear how medical evidence of your need will be sought. It is likely that you will be able to submit evidence from your own practitioner rather than having to be submitted to an independent assessment as was the case with the former Attendance and Mobility Allowances and self-assessment will be accepted at the discretion of the adjudicator.

The adjudication system involves a lay adjudication officer in making the initial decision. If you are not happy with her decision you must request a review. A different adjudication officer will then assess your case and another decision will be issued. You can then request further reviews. If you are unhappy with the review decision, you can appeal to the Disability Appeal Tribunal. Difficult medical questions may be referred by the adjudication officer to a Disability Allowance Advisory Board.

Existing claimants of Attendance Allowance or Mobility Allowance are protected in that they should be able to retain the right to claim benefit under their existing claims until the current expiry date.

**Disability Working Allowance (DWA)**  This is a completely new benefit being offered to people who have a disability and are working but earning a low wage. The amount of DWA available will be calculated in a similar way to Family Credit. The difference is that Family Credit is only available to working adults with responsibilities for children.

The DWA will be available to any disabled adults who can show that they are disabled and provide proof of receiving qualifying benefits for at least one day of 56 days before the claim of DWA, and that they are at a disadvantage in getting work. The benefit is also means-tested and only available for claimants who work more than 16 hours per week.

If you have capital over a certain amount you will not be eligible for this benefit. A DWA award is made for six months and the first claim is based on self-assessment unless the adjudication officer has reason to doubt the claimant's assessment. After six months the onus will be on the claimant to renew her application. Confirmation of disability will be required in subsequent claims. Receipt of Disability Living Allowance at the higher rate for mobility or one of the two higher rates for the care component, *or* receipt of Severe Disablement Allowance immediately before a DWA claim may be sufficient. Other claimants may be required to give information about their disability such as a list of functional disabilities which put them at a disadvantage in the job market. They may also be asked to nominate a professional (such as a GP, hospital doctor, community nurse, occupational psychologist, physiotherapist or occupational therapist) to give an assessment of their abilities. In rare cases it is envisaged that an independent assessment will be asked for by the adjudication officer.

## Benefits available to carers

**Invalid Care Allowance (ICA)**  ICA is a benefit paid to those who are not able to work because they are caring for a friend or relative who has a disability. The person you are caring for must be in receipt of Attendance Allowance or the middle or higher rate care component of the Disability Living Allowance. If you get ICA the person you are caring for is excluded from claiming Severe Disability Premium. You must be spending at least 35 hours per week caring for a person who qualifies. You must be aged between 16 and 60 (women) or 16 and 65 (men). Married women qualify for this allowance even if their husband is working. You must not be working or in full-time education although earnings from part-time work up to a certain limit are allowed. (The DSS can advise on the current limits.)

People receiving ICA are entitled to 12 weeks 'off' in any six month period. However, if the person you are caring for ceases to receive the qualifying allowance your 12 week entitlement may be shortened.

## General benefits

**Income Support** This benefit is payable to those who earn no income, or whose income is so low that they are considered to be eligible for 'topping up' from Income Support. To qualify you must be 18 or older (or 16–17 and pass other tests), you must not be in full-time, non-advanced education, you must not be working more than 24 hours per week, your partner (if you have one) must not be working for more than 24 hours per week, you must be available for work, actively seeking work or unable to work on account of caring responsibilities (for example looking after young children or disabled dependants) or due to incapacity for work. Children with severe disabilities who are unlikely to get a job may claim Income Support, while still at school, between the ages of 16 and 19. Capital savings over a certain limit will be counted against anyone making a claim for Income Support.

Certain other benefits are not counted as income if you apply for Income Support. These include Disability Living Allowance. If you are in receipt of ICA, Disability Living Allowance, Invalidity Benefit, Severe Disablement Allowance or are registered blind you should be entitled to a disability premium on top of your Income Support. If you are a single parent you should also receive an extra allowance. An element may be included within your Income Support known as the Carer's Premium (if you are receiving ICA or the Disabled Child's Premium otherwise).

**Child Benefit** This is an allowance paid to all carers of children who are 16 or under or, if older, still in full-time education. If you claim Income Support your Child Benefit will be deducted from the Income Support.

**Housing Benefit and help with Community Charge** If you are in receipt of Income Support or on a low income you may be eligible for Housing Benefit through which your local authority will pay some or all of your housing costs. You may also be entitled to payment of up to 80 per cent of your Community Charge bill (poll tax). You will be required to meet 20 per cent of Community Charge bills, all of water rates and house maintenance and insurance costs whatever your circumstances. If you are a house owner you may receive Income Support to enable you to pay interest on your mortgage but not the mortgage payments themselves.

There are certain instances where you are not entitled to Housing Benefit but where Income Support will cover your costs (such as rent and ground rent under a long tenancy and payments under a crown tenancy). Application forms for these benefits should be sought from your local authority (in respect of Housing Benefit and Community Charge Benefit) and from the Department of Social Security (in respect of Income Support).

Ownership of a certain amount of capital will be counted against claimants.

**The Social Fund** There are two types of social fund. Social Fund I gives a legal entitlement to maternity payment, funeral expenses and cold weather payments if certain conditions are met. Social Fund II is a discretionary loan or grant for which you can apply for certain essential items such as extra bedding or heating. The Social Fund is administered by local Social Security Offices under a budget system. Each office is allocated a budget and you will not be likely to be able to get access to a loan or grant if the budget for your area has been used up.

Capital savings over a certain amount count against claimants.

**Statutory Sick Pay (SSP)** This is usually payable for up to 28 weeks. If you are still sick after this period SSP is usually replaced by Invalidity Benefit. Unemployed and self-employed people are not covered by SSP and need to apply for Sickness Benefit instead – see below.

**Sickness Benefit** This is a benefit for people who are incapable of work because they are sick or disabled. It is payable for the first 28 weeks where you do not qualify for SSP. In order to qualify for Sickness Benefit, you need to have paid National Insurance contributions during the qualifying period, usually a set number of weeks of the preceding tax year to your claim. You must also have been incapable of work for more than three days in a row. If there is less than an eight week gap between these periods the qualifying period does not apply. You can earn up to a certain amount per week in addition to receiving sick pay if your doctor thinks that it is advisable for you to engage in some work. This benefit increases if you have dependants.

For the first week of sickness you can 'self-certificate'. After this period you need a certificate from your doctor confirming that you are unable to work due to sickness.

**Invalidity Benefit** This is a contributionary benefit (i.e. dependent on your National Insurance contributions) which may be available to people who have been incapable of work for a period of 28 weeks or more due to sickness or disability. Some other benefits and earnings are taken into account when a claim for Invalidity Benefit is assessed. The earnings disregard is more generous than for any other benefit. You may not be able to claim additions for dependants if they are earning money. You are allowed to earn a certain amount per week if your doctor considers that a limited amount of work will be of therapeutic benefit to you. If you are able to consistently work part-time you may be considered fit for work by the adjudication officer and your benefit stopped.

**Severe Disablement Allowance** This is a weekly cash benefit for people who have been incapable of work for at least 28 weeks and who do not have enough National Insurance contributions to qualify for Sickness and Invalidity Benefit. Alternative ways of qualifying for Severe Disablement Allowance are through entitlement to Attendance Allowance/Mobility Allowance/Disability Living Allowance, and incapacity for work prior to your 20th birthday. In addition you have to prove that you are 75–80 per cent disabled and have been so for at least 28 weeks. You should not automatically be excluded if you are in full-time education. However, the adjudication officer may decide that you are capable of work if you are able to be in full-time education.

Disablement is assessed by three criteria:

- Loss of faculty (this is any pathological condition or loss of the normal physical or mental function of a part of the body);
- Disability (this means an inability to perform a normal bodily or mental process);
- Disablement (this is the sum total of all the separate disabilities you may have – i.e. your overall inability to perform the normal activities of life).

There are guidelines which prescribe degrees of disability which are used to assess your eligibility under the 75–80 per cent rule (see *The Disability Rights Handbook*); also, an *SDA Handbook* is available from the DSS leaflet unit).

**Vaccine damage payments**   This scheme provides a tax free lump sum to people who are severely disabled as a result of vaccine damage. This includes people disabled because of vaccines given to their mothers prior to their birth.

**Grants from voluntary organisations**   There is a large number of voluntary organisations who are able to consider providing one-off grants for specific purposes.

The Royal National Institute for the Blind makes automatic grants to visually impaired children entering full-time, further or higher education or studying for Open University degrees.

## Practical help in the home

There are a number of sources from which practical help in the home may be available. Your local Social Services Department should be able to direct you to your local source of service provision. Some provision is made directly by Social Services or the local Health Service; other help is available from voluntary organisations and privately.

Standard services which may be available to you include the following:

- **Care Attendant Scheme** – which is aimed at helping disabled and elderly people to stay in the community. If there is no local scheme Crossroads Care run a national care attendant scheme. Under this scheme trained helpers can come into the home for specified periods to assist disabled people or provide respite for carers of disabled people.

- **District Nursing** – trained nurses can come into the home for specific tasks such as helping disabled people with dressing and washing.
- **Good Neighbour Scheme** – less formal than the care attendant scheme; volunteers are not necessarily trained.
- **Health visitors** – trained nurses able to come into the home to offer health care advice.
- **Home helps** – domestic helpers who can come into the home to help with cleaning and other light domestic tasks.
- **Homemaker scheme** – volunteers who can take over when your carer is ill so that you can be properly looked after at home.
- **Laundry service** – normally run by the Social Services Department (where one is available at all); collecting soiled sheets, bedding, clothes and nappies and returning them laundered.
- **Support for carers** – contact the National Carers Association for support and advice.
- **Meals on wheels** – provides a hot meal to your door on a regular basis.
- **Free nappies and aids to incontinence** – some local authorities provide nappies free of charge to children over the age of 2 who have disabilities. For older people who are incontinent, incontinence pads should also be available free of charge. Advice should be sought from your health visitor or from Social Services.

For some services, local authorities are empowered to recover charges from recipients who have sufficient means but they are not empowered to withdraw the service if you cannot pay.

## Help with equipment

Under the Chronically Sick and Disabled Persons Act 1970, the local authority has a duty to provide equipment for daily living, to help disabled people living in their own homes. This includes items which make it easier to use the toilet, to wash and dress etc.

An NHS consultant may prescribe any piece of equipment which he considers is necessary as part of a patient's treatment.

Wheelchairs (including powered chairs) and hand and pedal

controlled tricycles are supplied and maintained free of charge to a disabled person whose need for such a chair is permanent. Powered wheelchairs for occupant control out of doors are not available free of charge although there are loan schemes available through such organisations as Motability.

Electrical equipment to enable disabled individuals to control their environment (such as electrical appliances in the home) can be made available through the Department of Health.

'Possum' typewriters can be provided through the Local Educational Authority or employment service for use in school or the workplace. The local Department of Social Services should be consulted about such appliances for use in the home.

## Help outside the home

- **Adult Education** – see Chapter 8.
- **Employment schemes** – see Chapter 8.
- **Day hospital care** – this can be arranged for daytimes, allowing you to return home for nights on a regular basis, or just for emergencies.
- **Respite care, holiday, short-term care** – this can be provided by individual foster families or by residential centres and hospitals. It is primarily a service to enable carers to get a break.
- **Social and leisure activities** – the local authority has a duty to ensure that people with disabilities are enabled access to leisure activities outside the home and help with travelling to these activities.
- **Housebound Association** – this is a volunteer scheme to transport people with disabilities who are housebound to regular social activities and meetings.
- **Medical Escort Scheme** – if you cannot travel to hospital etc. on your own, the British Red Cross can offer this service.

## Help with transport

### Using a car

**Help with buying a car** A useful reference book is *Motoring and Mobility for Disabled People* available from RADAR. The Mobility Advice Information Service (MAVIS) can also offer advice on the phone or by letter.

Motability and Aid Vehicle Supplies (AVS) can both offer

help with purchasing second-hand cars. This can be either for a car to drive yourself or for someone else to drive for you.

There is a scheme whereby you can give over the higher rate of the mobility component of your disabled living allowance to Motability in return for the rent of a car.

Motability is a government funded scheme which helps disabled people who receive the higher rate of disability living allowance towards leasing a car or buying a new or second-hand car, through a hire-purchase scheme. They will loan you a certain sum of money which you then repay with your mobility allowance at a competitive rate of interest. For some people, particularly those needing expensive adaptations to their cars, this may not be enough to get them on the road and they will have to raise funds for the extra amount needed themselves.

**Exemption from road tax**  If you receive Disability Living Allowance (mobility component) and, possibly, if you have an Orange Badge, you may be eligible for vehicle tax exemption. This is providing the car is only for the use of the person for whom the benefit is received.

In order to be eligible for this exemption the beneficiary must have the car registered in her name. It is possible to register a car in joint names, and this might be most appropriate if the tax exemption is for a child. In addition you need to apply to your local vehicle registration office for an exception certificate. Form DLA403 to claim for this can be obtained from: Disability Living Allowance, Warbreck House, Warbreck Hill, Blackpool, FY2 OYE.

**Relief from VAT and car tax**  This applies to vehicles which are designed, or substantially and permanently adapted, for the carriage of a disabled person in a wheelchair or on a stretcher and no more than five other people. RADAR and DVLC both produce fact sheets on this benefit.

**Rate relief on garages**  This is available on garages, carports or land used for parking if you are registered as physically disabled with your local Social Services.

**Insurance**  Some insurance companies add premiums for disabled people whereas others specialise in offering reasonable insurance plans for those who have disabilities. RADAR can give advice about this.

**The Orange Badge Scheme** This provides parking concessions for people with severe disabilities and blind people who travel as drivers or as passengers. To qualify you need to demonstrate that you have a permanent and substantial disability which causes you very considerable difficulty in walking (as certified by your GP or consultant) or be in receipt of the mobility component of the Disability Living Allowance. There is no official lower age limit. I have known of children of the age of 2 being considered eligible in some circumstances.

Badge holders may park free of charge without time limit on parking meters and for up to two hours on single or double yellow lines providing they are not causing an obstruction in doing so.

The Orange Badge Scheme exempts you from toll fares over certain bridges in the UK.

## Buses

Travelling by bus has become more difficult for people with disabilities since the withdrawal of the conductor service on many routes throughout the country. Some major towns are developing special buses on specific routes which cater for people with disabilities but these are few and far between and may involve long waits. Your local Transport Office can advise on facilities in your area.

**Fare concessions** Concessions on fares are usually decided by your local authority. You may be eligible for a free bus pass outside peak times or tokens which can be used on a wide range of public transport.

## Taxi cards

A number of local authorities offer substantial concessions on the cost of taxi fares. This differs from one authority to another. You normally qualify in a similar way to the qualification for an Orange Badge.

## Further information

There are many more concessions available on most forms of public transport. Further information is available from The Department of Transport in *A Guide to Transport for People with Disabilities*.

# 10

# The future

Attitudes towards people with disabilities are changing slowly. Cerebral palsy is often a visible disability and this contributes to the slow pace of change. Also the helping professions are still under the influence of old ideas that people with cerebral palsy are slow developers with a poor outlook for their lives. In reality this simply is not the case. Even when a child is severely affected there are endless ways to ensure that he lives a full and rich life in which he can receive respect and equal status. It is crucial that we stop underestimating children's abilities and potential, that we treat them like ordinary kids and give them every opportunity to live fully in the community. It is only in this way that they are likely to develop into full members of society with awareness of their place within it. There are a growing number of voluntary agencies dedicated to the improvement of the quality of life for people with disabilities and campaigning for an improvement in service provision. It is well worth making contact with such agencies so that you can draw support from them in the early years of your child's development.

What follows will probably say more about the future than any dry discussion. These are rough sketches of the lives of three people who have cerebral palsy. Their experiences are unique to them as individuals but each person has highlighted areas where they felt their personal progress was hindered by their disability as well as issues for which the disability had no relevance. Many readers will be concerned for their child's future. These three people's lives cannot hold any clue to your own child's future but I hope you can take heart (as they have), enjoy life and help your children to enjoy theirs.

## Jacqueline

Jacqueline was born in 1927 in the provinces near Bristol. An only child, two months premature, born with jaundice, she choked half an hour after birth and was taken from her mother. There were no incubators in those days, so she was wrapped in cotton wool, rubbed in oil rather than washed, and a bottle of brandy was kept at the bottom of the bed.

After an apparent recovery there was no more involvement with the medical profession until her mother expressed concern over her development. Eventually she was diagnosed as having 'club feet' and 'hammer toes'. She walked at 3 years. At the age of 5 she had operations to her heels (tendon transplants), and to stiffen her big toes. She then had medical gym until she was 12 years old. Everything had to be paid for in those days, so the medical gym was private.

After a year with a governess she was able to attend the local private primary school (mornings only) from the age of 7. She moved schools at the age of 8 owing to the family moving house, and attended the primary level of a big high school. The headmistress thought she would do better in a smaller school so she was sent to a smaller private school where she stayed until she was 12. She was verbally bullied but did not feel able to tell her parents. In fact the whole family was treated to verbal admonishment. Jacqueline can remember comments made in public criticising her mother. After another move to Lincolnshire she settled down in a local high school for the rest of her schooldays.

Jacqueline eventually rebelled against medical gym and special shoes etc. She decided she wanted to go to university and concentrate on intellectual matters. She took a history degree in 1949. When she was in her second year at college there was a first year student who had cerebral palsy who would go along to college dances. Jacqueline could not bring herself to go because she felt quite incompetent, but she also felt ashamed at not coping so well.

Before graduating Jacqueline decided she wanted to be an archivist. After attending an interview at an appropriate training school she was dissuaded from pursuing her application on account of the inaccessibility of record offices in old buildings and the hefty weight of the archive materials. She eventually decided on a post-graduate course as a librarian which involved some archive work as part of the course.

Throughout her education she felt she was socially a very shy person though this was not the case in class. She thinks this shyness was probably contributed to by her feelings about her disability.

When it came to applying for training jobs Jacqueline explained her disability as 'slight stiffness of the legs' as the club feet had been operated on. She was overjoyed to get three job offers and chose a job in a small history library which would enable her to put her degree to good use.

Looking back on it she doesn't know how she managed some of the physical work she had to undertake. She remembers having to carry parcels from her waist to her chin to the local post office. At the end of this post she received good references which would set her up for any future career.

At the age of 25 she managed to get in to the London Foot Hospital to see the surgeon who attended monthly to see feet which required more attention than was available through chiropody. After seeing her walking pattern and testing the reflexes in her feet the surgeon announced, 'You know you're spastic don't you?' She was surprised and asked if anything else needed to be done. He asked about her work life and concluded 'You've more or less cured yourself'. She feels she was lucky, Scope had just been founded; the condition was 'in fashion' and being reviewed in women's magazines; otherwise she would not have known what the word meant. She then rushed off to the University of London Library and found an entry in a medical dictionary which made no sense to her until she got to the description of what it felt like. Then she felt 'Why the hell hasn't anybody told me before?!'

From 1951 to 1982 she worked in a number of posts as assistant librarian which included a spell in France doing research work for the Institute of Education. The approach to the library she worked at in France was very difficult but by the end of three months she had mastered it. However, she was not able to transfer this ability to other similar situations. In 1982 she took advantage of an early retirement scheme so that she could concentrate on the thesis she is still completing.

In the early 1970s she became afraid of the steepest part of the hill local to her home. Her doctor prescribed valium to relax her and some physiotherapy at University College Hospital. She feels that fear may play a large part in preventing some of the physical activities she feels unable to undertake.

In the Autumn of 1976 Jacqueline began to feel more

shaky and her writing didn't seem good. She was admitted to hospital and operated on for a kink in her spinal cord. A crumbling disc was fused with bone from her right hip. She has felt much improved since this operation. About a year after her operation an old muscle strain recurred. At the end of her successful treatment she still had a vague unease and her physiotherapist cleverly realised that it was the beginning of a new stage of relaxation. She has continued to improve via various therapies and massage techniques.

Jacqueline has always felt that her condition was ambiguous. Because of the mildness of her cerebral palsy she was never sure whether she was disabled or non-disabled and felt some confusion over her role in life. She was brought up to face situations and get on with life and could never really discuss her feelings about disability with her parents. In one way she did 'get on with life' but in another there was always a constant measuring of herself against 'normal'. Jacqueline would never say she was tired on the job unless others were saying it too.

Jacqueline describes herself as a Victorian spinster with no sexual experience, and wonders if a partner would have helped her to relax more. As with the shyness she is not sure how much her disability contributed to this situation.

In 1986 she joined the Foundation for Conductive Education after seeing the TV programme *Standing up for Joe*.

Jacqueline has been attending psychology workshops in France and has begun to allow herself to talk about her anger which would have hurt her parents.

# Andrew

Andrew is 45 years old. He was born in Palestine of Polish parents and came to England at the age of 12. He was treated for various symptoms associated with ignorance of his condition and was eventually diagnosed as spastic quadriplegic at about the age of 4 or 5. He followed the common route of specialist consultants followed by special schools.

He spent five years at St Margaret's Special School 'riding around on a tricycle'. Later he attended the Thomas Delarue Special School. The Thomas Delarue was unusual amongst special schools for its emphasis on obtaining academic qualifications. Andrew felt there was a repressive atmosphere there and this, coupled with his own onrush of sudden personal development, led to him being regarded as disruptive, unco-operative and rebellious. Despite the low expectations of the school he managed to get 'O' and 'A' levels. Both of the schools he attended were boarding schools. He feels that they were effectively prisons so that opportunities to compare his experience with other, non-disabled people were only available by comparing himself with the staff who were the only non-disabled people he had contact with. He felt that there were set rules for his future against which he wanted to rebel.

> 'If people think you're clever and you're disabled you *have* to go to university. One reason for this is to continue to show that disabled people can be clever. The choice is limited because of the high expectation and the need to prove that disabled people can be clever whereas others might choose to go to university either to prepare for a career or simply to have a good time.'

Andrew decided against going to university. Instead, he went to the London College of Printing to study art. He had applied to go to the Hornsey College of Art (which was *the* place to go in the 1960s). They accepted him but the building didn't so he had to look around for a building that was accessible. The London College of Printing said that they were. However, the lifts did not service all floors, classes were held regularly in different buildings with 100 stairs in every part and there were regular visits to inaccessible museums. Andrew gave up after a year. The strain of coping with no support meant that he simply wasn't producing the required quantity of work.

He joined the GLC with the intention of short-term employment before returning to art college.

> '. . . and probably as 99 per cent of those who have done it would say "you never go back". The GLC was a good place to work from anyone's point of view. The place was buzzing and there was a dynamism and enthusiasm that I haven't felt since.'

A succession of local government jobs followed, the latest of which is the position of Access Officer for Camden Council.

Andrew feels that his abilities are neither appreciated nor used in local government positions. Everyone has to compromise during their career but Andrew feels that disability has forced him to compromise where he might otherwise have had the opportunity to earn money in his preferred field; one where his artistic abilities would have been made much more use of. He could have exercised the option not to work at all but to have gone off travelling and painting or he could have gone and worked on the Victoria line and made pots of money to enable him to carry on painting.

Looking back on it he can now see what should have happened:

- At school you find out what you probably want to do;
- At the point of choice research and negotiation takes place to ensure that proper support will be available.

Andrew has found it much easier to succeed in employment than in art college because the college atmosphere is very active and nothing in his special school equipped him to make the link between school and college. He has finally reached a point where he doesn't see anything wrong in asking for help and realising that it does not equal an admission of defeat. One problem about asking for help is knowing who the right person is to ask:

'For example, you're in your car and you need someone to get your chair out. You look at every single person walking towards you and you make judgements in an absurd way about who will and who won't help. So you wait and you wait. Then you say "Excuse me. Are you busy?" "Have you got a minute?" and the person you've picked hasn't got time or they've done their back in. What you need first and foremost is the confidence to ask. Assertiveness training for people with disabilities and their parents should be offered early enough to be useful to them.'

Andrew feels a conflict in doing a job as a disabled person which is strongly related to disability issues. On the one hand he questions whether he should be seen to be doing a job which appears to be a 'natural' for a disabled person while on the other hand he believes that only a disabled person could adequately do that job.

One of the high spots in Andrew's life, where the issue of his disability did not enter into it, was sharing a flat in Wimbledon when coincidentally, he was physically at his fittest. Andrew currently shares a house in London and also has his own house in the country where he retreats for weekends and holidays. It is here that he enjoys developing his other interest – woodwork.

Andrew's view on disadvantage and disability is that you *are* disadvantaged if you *feel* disadvantaged. You feel at a disadvantage either because of your own and other people's conditioning or because you may be so. Being told to learn to cope reinforces the view that you are at a disadvantage. He feels that the key to successful living as a person who has disabilities is organisation: 'I am disabled. I'm not totally happy about it, but I can organise my life around it.'

# Martin

Martin was born in 1963 and is one of six children. He was born in Haringay which is where he now lives in his own flat. He attended a local special school which was a day school:

> 'Special schools are disgusting because of the low expectations they have of the pupils. It makes you feel different just being there. It creates a "them and us" mentality. You know there is a world out there but you are not part of it. When you leave school you are stuck at home. The Christmas parties and charity events stop.'

Martin remembers one of his teachers saying to him, 'Everyone loves a child, but nobody's going to love you as an adult.' Martin is against charities such as 'Children in Need' because, he feels, they just throw money at people without changing the way the system treats people with disabilities. To make matters worse the money often goes to promote segregated activities.

Martin had plenty of opportunity to study academically but feels that the exam system is not geared for people with disabilities. At 16 he had the choice of staying on at school, getting a job or going to a college of further education. He chose to go to college and attended a residential college for people with disabilities in Cheltenham. He felt that this college was a grown up version of his special school. He studied art, English and sport. The one plus about college was that it did expect students to question themselves about independence.

While he was at college Martin tried to develop a physical relationship with different women, all fellow students. There was Shelley, who had spina bifida; Liz, with whom he fell heavily in love; and Lesley, who was going out with his best friend. He also became very fond of Caroline, a member of staff. During his time at college he got very depressed and made more than one suicide attempt. He sat at the edge of the lake and seriously contemplated this option but in the end something stopped him. All his male friends seemed to have girlfriends and he was the only one who didn't. At one of the end of term discos he thought his luck was in with Liz but it didn't come off. He spent the next six weeks thinking about her and believing she really cared but when he got back to college she avoided him.

'Sex education was something you found at the corner shop. I smuggled some magazines into college and got told off by the matron. The cleaner was disgusted with the posters I had on my wall.'

When Martin left college he was determined to get a place of his own. His mother's house was full of stairs. He didn't have a bedroom of his own. The doors were too narrow to take the wheelchair he sometimes uses and the bathroom was a nightmare. He contacted a social worker who put him in touch with the local council Housing Department. He didn't qualify. The council official who came round maintained that he was better off at home with his family and anyway he didn't score enough points. The social worker then put him in touch with Habinteg Housing Association who offer specially adapted housing for wheelchair users. He was told he would have a 10 year wait but he was lucky and a flat became available after 18 months. Martin has been living independently in his specially adapted flat for nine years.

Martin takes medication which helps him to relax and gets him pleasantly 'high' if mixed with alcohol. The drugs, Baclofen and Carisoms, make him tired but without them he gets tense and walking becomes difficult. He was refused relaxants when he asked for them at school. He did not take any drugs until he was 16 and the main reason he took the decision to accept drugs was so that he could relax. This enabled him to do more – for example, typing, operating videos and changing records. Martin finds that if he worries about the difficulty of a task it becomes even more difficult. The drugs help him to become more confident. He sometimes takes them to help him get a good night's sleep. They have become a lifeline which he can't live without. If he cuts down the dose it works for a couple of days but then he feels as if he is waking from a deep sleep and familiar feelings of tension creep back. The uncertainty of handling such objects as sausages and bacon returns.

Another issue he had to confront when he came home from college was that of his sexuality. Martin now realised that he had always been gay (although this might not have found expression if one of the girls at college had responded positively). His social worker was the first person outside the family that he told he was gay and she was very supportive. His younger sister was also supportive. He was living a double life at his mother's home. He tried to go to local youth clubs and be 'one of the lads'. He had to make a conscious effort to look at the girls when he really wanted to look at the guys. One night he made a 4 am call to Gay Switchboard and this was the turning point. Through this contact he got involved with a local group called 'Ice Breakers'. From there he got involved with another group called 'Help a London Friend'. He said he just wanted to 'put one foot in the water' and they said 'Fine'. Eventually, he got taken to various places and began to see a place which was alien to the one his family was brought up to believe in. The more he saw the more he liked it.

For work Martin started off on the community pro-gramme working with mentally handicapped people as a facilitator. Then, from 1985–1987 he worked at the Haringay Disability Association on a project called 'Jobability' as an administrative assistant. He points out that people with disabilities tend to get the lower level jobs in such organisations. Martin is currently unemployed but is developing his talents as a poet and writer. He is now beginning to do poetry readings and recently did a reading for the BBC.

Since he has been involved in the gay community he has been able to mix with like-minded people. Although he is still in the minority in terms of race and disability he has more of a sense of belonging and he feels that gay people are much more willing to accept you as you are. He gets depressed sometimes but then reminds himself that there must be thousands of people like him who have not been able to express themselves because they are repressed:

> 'Making decisions for *me* is the most important thing. Not the social workers or the disability organisations.'

The following poem written by Martin is based on his mother. He feels she had to go through so much pain and is still going through so much pain and it's not right that she should have to.

### Pain of a black woman

*I was walking along a dry and dusty road;*
*The sun shining with no respite;*
*With this scene, my tale starts to unfold;*
*A black woman came forward, eyes shining bright;*

*'What are you doing here', she asks, in her voice a hint of scorn*
*My answer – 'Good day ma'am, I'm here to greet the sunny beautiful morn;*
*I'm here to explore another world I've never seen before';*
*Her answer – 'Then I will tell you about my pain which seems to hurt*
*    more and more:*
*My health is suffering, the father of my children is dead,*
*I act so good and noble, knowing there is no flour left to make the bread;*
*The soldiers come, accusing my sons of plotting against their country;*
*I cried, let them be, you can't deny them their right to be home with me;*
*They told me to be quiet, to leave it alone;*
*I watched them with a heavy heart as they left me on my own;*
*I'm left with my baby daughter, there is no food here for us;*
*This is my country, the place of my birth, yet there is no one left to trust';*

*I never knew what it was like to suffer as this woman had;*
*I forgot my own troubles and held her in my arms;*
*I asked her what would she do;*
*Her answer – 'Survive and carry on until I cannot;*
*This is Africa, I cannot fight the prejudice;*
*Looking for what's right in a country where there is no justice;*
*Try being here, struggling to survive;*
*Try it just fighting to stay alive';*

*I knew I could not help her, but at least I was able to share the pain,*
*The pain of this incredible, marvellous black woman.*

# USEFUL ADDRESSES AND CONTACTS

## Organisations offering general advice and/or services to people who have cerebral palsy

### Scope
12 Park Crescent, London W1N 4EQ
Tel: 0171–636 5020

Offers a wide range of activities to help children and adults who have cerebral palsy including advice, research, holidays, residential care, education and training, assessment, support and information, publications and videos.

Scope's Cerebral Palsy Helpline, 0800 626216, is a free helpline offering information, advice and initial counselling on anything associated with cerebral palsy.

### London Boroughs Disability Resource Team
Third Floor, Bedford House, 125–133 Camden High Street, London NW1 7JR
Tel: 0171–482 5299

Provides specialist services and expertise to enable local authorities and public organisations to meet the needs of disabled people.

### Scottish Council on Disability
Information Department, 5 Shandwick Place, Edinburgh EH2 4RG
Tel: 0131–229 8632

Provides information to disabled people resident in Scotland and those working with them.

### Northern Ireland Information Service for Disabled People
2 Annadale Avenue, Belfast BT7 3JH
Tel: 01232 491011

A comprehensive information service, including aids with a Northern Ireland orientation.

# Support for parents in the early years

### Contact a Family
170 Tottenham Court Road, London W1P 0HA
Tel: 0171–383 3555

A national charity which supports families who have children with different disabilities or special needs. They aim to help families to overcome isolation by bringing them together through local mutual support and self-help groups.

CRY-SIS
BM CRY-SIS, London WC1N 3XX
Tel: 0171–404 5011

Support group for parents of crying babies.

### Parents Anonymous
6 Manor Gardens, London N7
Tel: 0171–263 8918

Support group for parents who fear they may batter their children.

### Carers' National Association
29 Chilworth Mews, London W2 3RG
Tel: 0171–490 8898

Umbrella organisation for carers' groups offering information, contacts, advice and support for anyone caring for an elderly, sick or disabled person at home.

### The National Childbirth Trust
Alexandra House, Oldham Terrace, London W3 6NH
Tel: 0181–992 8637

Offers support and information to parents during pregnancy and the early years of parenthood. Resources include antenatal teaching, breast feeding counsellors and many local postnatal support networks.

# Treatment and therapy

## College of Speech Therapists
Harold Poster House, 6 Lechmere Road, London NW2 5BU
Tel: 0171–459 8521

Provides pamphlets for parents and can advise on the location of qualified speech therapists.

## The Kerland Clinic
Marsh Lane, Huntworth Gate, Bridgwater, Somerset TA6 6LQ
Tel: 01278 429089

Private clinic offering assessment and treatment based on the ideas of Doman Delacato. Aims to offer a less intensive but equally effective treatment to many similar clinics.

## BIRD (Brain Injury Rehabilitation Development, Centre for)
The BIRD centre, 131 Main Road, Broughton, Chester CH4 0NR
Tel: 01244 532047

A treatment centre employing unique approaches developed by the centre to inhibit primitive reflexes and provide for normal functional ability. The methods are relevant to the full age and severity range of brain injury victims. The centre was featured on BBC's *How do they do that?* in 1994.

## British Institute for Brain Damaged Children (BIBDC)
Knowle Hall, Knowle, Bridgwater, Somerset
Tel: 01278 684060

Private centre offering assessment and treatment based on the ideas of Doman Delacato.

## The Bobath Centre
250 East End Road, London W2 8AU
Tel: 0181–444 3355

Bobath centres have now opened up in Wales and Scotland.

Scotland: Tel: 0141 9502922

Wales: Tel: 01222 522600

## The British Society for Music Therapy
69 Avonlea Avenue, East Barnet, Herts EN4 8NB
Tel: 0181–368 8879

Promotes the use of music therapy in the treatment and education of adults and children who have disabilities.

## The Nordoff Robbins Music Therapy Centre
3 Leighton Place, London NW5 2QL

Offers courses for teachers and therapists interested in music therapy, especially with regard to severely disabled and brain damaged children.

## The British Association of Art Therapy
13c Northwood Road, London N6 5LT

Professional association for art therapists.

## Vibro Acoustics
Kirton Products, 23 Rookwood Way, Haverhill,
Suffolk CB9 8PA
Tel: 01440 705352

This is the company which markets vibro acoustic therapy equipment. Vibro acoustics provide relief from tension caused by stress, pain and spastic conditions.

## Physiotherapy and Music Therapy Department
Harperbury Hospital, Harper Lane, Radlett WD7 9HQ

This department is carrying out research into the use of vibro acoustic therapy.


# Communication and aids for daily living

## Scottish Centre of Technology for the Communication Impaired
Victoria Infirmary, Langside, Glasgow

Provides Scotland-wide assessments, training and information for professionals and participates in research and development in communication difficulty and technology.

## REMAP
25 Mortimer Street, London W1N 8AB

Offers engineering help for the disabled by making 'one-off' aids for individuals whose needs cannot be met by standard commercial aids or appliances.

**Disabled Living Foundation**
380/384 Harrow Road, London W9 2HU
Tel: 0171–289 6111

Works to find non-medical solutions to the daily living problems facing disabled people of all ages. The DLF's main activities are research and information provision.

**The Communication Advice Centre**
Musgrave Park Hospital, Stockman's Lane, Belfast BT9 7JB
Tel: 01232 669501 ext. 561

A centre specially staffed and equipped with many of the aids available to help patients with communication disorders offering practical demonstrations and individual advice on specific problems.

**Genesis Orthotics Limited**
1 Holt Court, Off Jennens Road, Aston Science Park,
Birmingham B7 4EJ
Tel: 0121 359 5717

Genesis Orthotics are now the distributers for the David Hart walker. At this centre children can be assessed for the use of these walkers and an after care service is available to ensure that the walker is adapted as necessary with the child's growth.

**G. & S. Smirthwaite**
16 Daneheath Business Park, Heathfield, Newton Abbott,
Devon TQ12 6TL
Tel: 01626 835552

Suppliers of aids and equipment.

**Ace Centre**
Omerod School, Waynfleet Road, Headington, Oxford
Tel: 01865 63508

Offers assessment for communication aids in the southern half of England. The northern counterpart is on 0161 627 1358.

**Facilitated Communication**
Tel: 0171–433 1146

Information about facilitated communication in the UK.

# Alternative/complementary treatments

**The British Acupuncture Association and Register**
34 Alderney Street, London SW1V 4EU
Tel: 0171–834 1012/6229

Publishes a handbook of practitioners.

**The British Homoeopathic Association**
27a Devonshire Street, London W1N 1RJ
Tel: 0171–935 2163

**The Tisserand Aromatherapy Institute**
10 Victoria Grove, Second Avenue, Hove, East Sussex BN3 2LJ
Tel: 01273 206640

Can advise on training courses and weekend seminars and have a list of qualified therapists.

**The International Federation of Aromatherapists**
Department of Continuing Education, Royal Masonic Hospital, Ravenscourt Park, London W6 0TN
Tel: 0181–846 8066

**The Association of Reflexologists**
27 Old Gloucester Street, London WC1 3XX

Send a large stamped addressed envelope for information.

**The General Council and Register of Osteopaths**
1 Suffolk Street, London SW1Y 4HG
Tel: 0171–839 2060

**Herbal Medicine Association**
PO Box 304, Bournemouth, Dorset BH7 6JZ
Tel: 01202 433691

# Support in caring

**Community Service Volunteers**
237 Pentonville Road, London N1 9NJ
Tel: 0171–278 6601

Volunteer scheme to support people with disabilities with independent living and to offer general assistance.

**Crossroads Care Attendant Scheme**
10 Regent Place, Rugby, Warwickshire CV21 2PN
Tel: 01788 73653

Practical help for limited periods for families with a disabled member.


# Legal advice

**Action for Victims of Medical Accidents**
Bank Chambers, 1 London Road, Forest Hill, London SE23 3TP
Tel: 0171–291 2793

Offers advice to people considering taking legal action against the health authority for medical negligence.


# Education

**The Hornsey Centre for Children Learning**
26A Dukes Avenue, Muswell Hill, London N10 2PT
Tel: 0181–444 7241/2

A centre which offers early education programmes based on conductive education.

**The Foundation for Conductive Education**
The National Institute of Conductive Education, Cannon Hill House, Russell Road, Mosely, Birmingham B13 8RD

An organisation providing conductive education in this country replicating the methods taught at the Peto Institute in Hungary. Also has further information on conductive education in other parts of the UK.

**Advisory Centre for Education (ACE) Ltd**
Unit 1B, Aberdeen Studios, 22–24 Highbury Grove,
London N5 2EA
Tel: 0171–354 8321

A registered charity offering free advice, service and publications for parents with a focus on school years (5–18) in Local Education Authority schools only. They can advise on many questions parents might have about their children's educational rights and publish very useful and easy to read guides to the law in this area.

## Children's Legal Centre
20 Compton Terrace, London N1 2UN
Tel: 0171–359 6251

Gives information and advice on all aspects of the law affecting children, including The Education Act 1981.

## Parents for Inclusion (formerly Parents in Partnership)
Unit 2, Ground floor, 70 South Lambeth Road,
London SW8 1RL
Tel: 0171–735 7735

Working for inclusive educational opportunities for children with special needs. Has a number of local groups.

## National Portage Association
King Alfred's College, Sparkford Road, Winchester,
Hants SO22 4NR
Tel: 01962 62281

Provides teams of advisers who work with parents of pre-school children in their home to support early learning. Can provide details of local schemes.

## National Bureau for Handicapped Students
40 Brunswick Square, London WC1N 1AZ
Tel: 0171–278 3459/3450

Has a range of useful information and literature about further education.

## Open University
Undergraduate Admissions Office, PO Box 48,
Milton Keynes MK7 6AN

## Queen Elizabeth's Foundation for the Disabled
Leatherhead, Surrey, KT22 0BN
Tel: 01372 84 2204

Has four centres which provide assessment, further education, vocational training, residential sheltered work, holidays and convalescence.

## Rudolph Steiner House
35 Park Road, London NW1 6XT
Tel: 0171–723 8219

**Camphill Village Trust**
Delrow House, Hilfield Lane, Aldenham, Watford,
Herts WD2 8DJ
Tel: 01923 856006

**The Human Scale Education Movement**
96 Carlingcott, Near Bath, Avon BA2 8AW
Tel: 01761 433733

**Education Otherwise**
Tel: 01891 518303

**Montessori Nursery and Pre-School Information Line**
Tel: 0171–224 5080

**Montessori Primary and Secondary Information Line**
Tel: 0171–487 4342

## Housing and environment

**National Federation of Housing Associations**
175 Grays Inn Road, London WC1
Tel: 0171–278 6571

**The Housing Corporation**
Waverley House, Noel Street, London W1
Tel: 0171–434 2161

**SHAD (Sheltered Housing Assistance for the Disabled)**
c/o Battersea Arts Centre, Old Town Hall, Lavender Hill,
London SW11 5TF
Tel: 0171–350 1721

Aims to facilitate independent living schemes for severely
disabled people.

**Derbyshire Centre for Independent Living**
Victoria Buildings, 117 High Street, Clay Cross, Chesterfield,
Derbyshire
Tel: 01246 865305

Aims to provide care attendants to enable independent living.

**Hampshire Centre for Independent Living**
c/o John Evans, Le Court, Liss, Hampshire GU35 6HD

A scheme devised to help severely disabled people to find
alternative accommodation and support outside residential
care.

**BCOP (British Council of Organisations of Disabled People)**
c/o Yeoman's House, 76 St James's Lane, Muswell Hill,
London N10

Aims to involve disabled people in planning for their individual housing needs to be met.

**Centre on Environment for the Handicapped**
126 Albert Street, London NW1 7NF
Tel: 0181–482 2247

Provides a specialist information and advisory service on the environmental needs of people with disabilities.

**Shelter**
88 Old Street, London EC1
Tel: 0171–253 0202

**British Standards Institute**
Sales Department, 101 Pentonville Road, London N1 9DR
Tel: 0171–837 8801

# Support for people who have disabilities in addition to cerebral palsy

**SENSE**
311 Grays Inn Road, London WC1X 8PT
Tel: 0171–278 1000

Offers a wide range of services for parents of children who have dual sensory impairment including educational advice, training, information, support and advice.

**Twins with Special Needs**
10 Tolpuddle Way, Yateley, Camberley, Surrey, GU17 7BH

**Royal National Institute for the Blind**
224 Great Portland Street, London W1N 6AA
Tel: 0171–388 1266

Runs schools and educational advisory services, colleges, courses, publications, aids and equipment.

**MENCAP (Royal Society for Mentally Handicapped Children and Adults)**
117/123 Golden Lane, London EC1Y 0RT
Tel: 0171–253 9433

The major organisation for parents of children and adults with learning difficulties. Many local affiliated branches.

**Royal National Institute for the Deaf**
105 Gower Street, London WC1E 6AH
Tel: 0171–387 8033

## Specialist dentists

The local District Dental Officer in the Community Dental Service (will be in your local phone book) should have information on specialist services in your locality.

The British Society of Dentistry for the Handicapped is a national organisation which meets regularly to discuss the dentistry needs of people with special needs. The address changes from year to year but is currently:

The Honorary Secretary
Dr J. H. Nunn
Dept of Child Dental Health, The Dental School, Framlington Place, Newcastle upon Tyne NE2 4BW

## Pressure groups

**British Council of Disabled People (BCODP)**
Litchurch Plaza, Litchurch Lane, Derby DE24 8AA
Tel: 01332 295 551

An umbrella group for local and specific interest pressure groups run by and for people with disabilities.

**People First**
Instrument House, 207–215 Kings Cross Road,
London WC1X 9DB
Tel: 0171–713 6400

A self-advocacy organisation run by and for people with learning difficulties.

**The Alliance for Inclusive Education** (formerly the Integration Alliance)
Unit 2, Ground Floor, 70 Lambeth Road, London SW8 1RL
Tel: 0171–735 5277

An organisation which lobbies for and offers information about inclusive education.


# Organisations for people who may be subjected to further discrimination

**Community Health Groups for Ethnic Minorities (CHGEM)**
28 Churchfield Road, London W3 6EB
Tel: 0171–993 6119

An independent national charity which aims to resolve some of the health and social problems that arise in ethnic communities. Offers basic advice and interpreting and translating services for health care workers.

**Ethnic Switchboard**
2B Lessingham Avenue, London SW17 8LU
Tel: 0171–682 0216/7

**Gay Men's Disabled Group**
c/o Gay's the Word, 66 Marchmont Street, London WC1N 1AB

Aims to provide support to gay men with disabilities and to bring gay men with and without disabilities together.

**Gemma\***
BM Box 5700, London WC1N 3XX

A group for disabled and non-disabled lesbians aiming to lessen the isolation of those whose disability might hinder appropriate relationships.

**Gay and Lesbian Switchboard**
BM Switchboard, London WC1
Tel: 0171–837 7324

24 hour information and help.

**Childline**
FREEPOST, London EC4B 4BB
Tel: 0171–239 1000

(Free telephone helpline for children needing support – 0800 1111)

# Adult life

**Remploy Ltd**
415 Edgware Road, Cricklewood, London NW2 6LR
Tel: 0181–452 8020

Employs severely disabled people in factories throughout Britain.

**SPOD (Society to Aid Personal and Sexual Relationships of Disabled People)**
286 Camden Road, London N7 0BJ
Tel: 0171–607 8851

**Disdate**
56 Devizes Avenue, Bedford
Tel: 01234 40643

Penfriend/dating agency for disabled people and for lonely people.

**The Outsiders Club**
Box 4ZB, London W1A 4ZB
Tel: 0171–741 3332

Aims to rescue people who have become emotionally stranded because of difference.

**British Sports Association for the Disabled**
34 Osnaburgh Street, London NW1 3ND
Tel: 0171–383 7277

# FURTHER READING

**Medical**
Parish, Peter (1987) *Medicines: A Guide for everybody*. Penguin.
Jepson, Marion E. (1983) *Community Child Health*. Hodder and
  Stoughton.

**Alternative medicine**
Grossman, Richard (1986) *The Other Medicines*. Pan.
Hulk, Malcolm (1978) *The Encylopaedia of Alternative Medicine
  and Self Help*. Rider.

**Physiotherapy**
Cotton, Ester *The Basic Motor Pattern*. The Spastics Society.
Cotton, Ester *The Hand as a Guide to Learning*. The Spastics
  Society.
Finnie, Nancie R. (1989) *Handling the Young Cerebral Palsied
  Child at Home*. Heinemann Medical.
Levitt, Sophie (1982) *Treatment of Cerebral Palsy and Motor Delay*.
  Blackwell Scientific.
Levitt, Sophie (1984) *Paediatric Development Therapy*. Blackwell
  Scientific.

**Speech and language therapy**
McConkey, Roy and Penny Price *Let's Talk*. Human Horizon.
Warner, Jennifer *Helping the Handicapped Child with Early
  Feeding*. Winslow Press.

**Conductive education**
Cotton, Phillipa J. and Andrew Sutton *Conductive Education: A
  System for Overcoming Motor Disorder*. Chapman Hall.
Hari, Maria and Karoly Akos (1988) *Conductive Education*
  (Translated from Hungarian). Routledge.

**Patterning**
Baker, Margaret and Trevor England *Don't Learn to Live with It*.
  Holywell Press. Available from The Kerland Clinic.
Cummins, Robert A. (1988) *The Neurologically Impaired Child:
  Doman Delacato Techniques Reappraised*. Croom Helm.

Hunter, Ian (1987) *Brain Injury: Tapping the Potential Within.* Ashgrove Press.

Scotson, Linda *Doran. Child of Courage.* Pan.

## Guides for parents

Scope. *Your Child has Cerebral Palsy.* Parent Information Pack.

Clarke, P., H. Kofsky and J. Lauroi (1989) *To a Different Drumbeat: A Practical Guide to Parenting Children with Special Needs.* Hawthorn Press.

Griffiths, Margaret and Mare Clegg (1988) *Cerebral Palsy: Problems and Practice.* Souvenir Press.

Nancy, Kohner (1988) *Caring at Home.* The Kings Fund.

Murray, Pippa and Jill Penman (1996) *Let our Children be.* Published by Parents with Attitude, c/o 44 Cowlishaw Road, Sheffield S11 8XF.

Wilson, Judy *Caring Together: Guidelines for Carers' Self-Help and Support Groups.* The National Extension College.

Worthington, Ann (1989) *Useful Addresses for Parents with a Handicapped Child.* Available from Ann Worthington, 10 Norman Road, Sale, Cheshire, M33 3DF

## Pre-school

Freeman, Joan (1991) *Bright as a Button: How to Encourage your Children's Talents 0–5 Years.* Optima. (This book was written with the unusually gifted child in mind; however, the play ideas in it are excellent and can be applied to any child.)

Matterson, E. M. (1975) *Play with a Purpose for Under-Sevens.* Penguin.

Sheridan, Mary (1977) *Spontaneous Play in Early Childhood, from Birth to Six Years.* NFER-Nelson Company Ltd.

## Education

*ACE Summary of the 1981 Education Act.* Published by ACE.

*Under 5s with Special Needs.* Published by ACE.

Haskell, Simon H. and Elizabeth K. Barrett (1989) *The Education of Children with Motor and Neurological Disabilities.* Chapman and Hall.

Hope, Mary (1984) *Micros for Children with Special Needs.* Blackwell Scientific.

Rieser, Richard and Micheline Mason (1990) *Disability Equality in the Classroom: A Human Rights Issue.* Published by Disability Equality in Education, 78 Mildmay Grove, London N1 4PJ.

## Housing
Rostron, John *Housing for the Physically Disabled*. Published by Liverpool Polytechnic.

## Adult life
ASBAH *Sex for Young People with Spina Bifida or Cerebral Palsy*. ASBAH with the co-operation of Scope.

Craft, Michael and Ann Craft *Handicapped Married Couples*. Routledge.

Greengross, Wendy *Entitled to Love: The Sexual and Emotional Needs of the Handicapped*. From SPOD.

Nordqvist, Inger *Life Together*. Available from the Royal Association for Disability and Rehabilitation, 25 Mortimer St, London W1N 8AB.

Rowntree Memorial Trust *After 16 – What Next?* The Family Fund, Joseph Rowntree Memorial Trust.

## Legal rights and benefits
Darnbrough, Ann and Derek Kinrade (1985) *Directory for Disabled People*. Woodhead-Faulkner. Has a comprehensive section on sport and leisure.

Disability Alliance. *Disability Rights Handbook*. A new edition is produced annually in April by the Disability Alliance ERA.

## Politics of disability
Longley, Susan (1990) *Women and Disability*. Macmillan.

Bryan, Joanna and Frank Thomas (1987) *The Politics of Mental Handicap*. Free Association Books.

## Fiction and autobiography
Southall, Ivan (1968) *Let the Balloon Go*. Puffin

Horwood, William (1988) *Skallagrigg*. Penguin.

Brown, Christy (1989) *My Left Foot*. Mandarin.

Nolan, Christopher (1987) *Under the Eye of the Clock*. Weidenfeld & Nicolson.

## Books for children
Pettenuzzo, Brenda and Maria Hill (1988) *I Have Cerebral Palsy*. Franklin Watts.

Scope have a fairly comprehensive bookshop and a booklist can be obtained by contacting their Library and Information Unit.

# INDEX

# Understanding Your Hyperactive Child

### The essential guide for parents

## Professor Eric Taylor

What is the difference between a high spirited child and one who is hyperactive? What are the causes? Can it be controlled? Can diet make a difference? These are just some of the issues addressed by Eric Taylor in the updated version of his book for the parents of hyperactive children.

# The Down's Syndrome Handbook

### A practical guide for families and carers

## Dr Richard Newton
## with The Down's Syndrome Association

Written and published in conjunction with The Down's Syndrome Association, by a doctor with a Down's syndrome child, this is a practical and realistic guide to coping with and caring for a Down's child.

# Living With Schizophrenia

### A positive guide for sufferers and carers

## Dr Brenda Lintner

Schizophrenia is a major mental illness which affects the entire personality and is commonly misunderstood. However schizophrenia can respond to treatment, and this practical and sympathetic guide is a source of vital information for all those concerned.

# Diabetes: The Complete Guide

## The essential introduction to managing diabetes

## Dr Rowan Hillson

Confronting a diagnosis of diabetes can be a frightening, confusing and depressing experience. This authoritative, comprehensive guide show how life with diabetes can be fulfilling and enjoyable.

# Reflexology

## An introductory guide to its uses

## Anya Gore

A form of therapy dating back thousands of years, reflexology can help in the treatment of a wide rang of illnesses but is particularly good for stress-related problems. This book concentrates on the experience from the client's viewpoint and answers the most frequently asked questions in a practical and straightforward way.

# Aromatherapy

## An introductory guide to professional and home use

## Gill Martin, with a foreword by Anita Roddick

An aromatherapy massage can be pure indulgence - or an effective way to help overcome common aliments. The oils can be used to help you relax and unwind or can be chosen to invigorate the body after a long and tiring day. This valuable and straightforward guide answers the common questions often asked about the history and theory of aromatherapy, including what to expect from a visit to an aromatherapist and the cost and availability of treatment.

To order your copy direct (p&p free), use the form below or call TBS DIRECT on **01621 819596**.

Please send me

... copies of **UNDERSTANDING YOUR HYPERACTIVE CHILD** @ £8.99 each

... copies of **THE CEREBRAL PALSY HANDBOOK** @ £9.99 each

... copies of **LIVING WITH SCHIZOPHRENIA** @ £8.99 each

... copies of **DIABETES: THE COMPLETE GUIDE** @ £8.99 each

... copies of **REFLEXOLOGY** @ £5.99 each

... copies of **AROMATHERAPY** @ £6.99 each

Mr/Ms/Mrs/Miss/ Other (Block Letters)

....................................................................................................................

Address:.........................................................................................................

....................................................................................................................

....................................................................................................................

Postcode:..................................Signed:.........................................

## HOW TO PAY

☐ I enclose a cheque/postal order for £................. made payable to 'TIPTREE BOOK SERVICES'

☐ I wish to pay by Access/Visa/Switch/Delta card

(delete where appropriate)

Card Number: ☐☐☐☐☐☐☐☐☐☐☐☐☐☐

Expiry Date: ☐☐☐☐

Post order to **TBS Direct, Tiptree Book Services, St. Lukes Chase, Tiptree, Essex, CO5 0SR.**

POSTAGE AND PACKING ARE FREE. Offer open in Great Britain including Northern Ireland. Books should arrive less than 28 days after we receive your order; they are subject to availability at time of ordering. If not entirely satisfied return in the same packaging and condition as received with a covering letter within 7 days. Vermilion books are available from all good booksellers.